Arthritis

A self-help guide to feeling better

Wendy Green

Foreword by Susan Oliver, nurse advisor to the
National Rheumatoid Arthritis Society

PERSONAL HEALTH GUIDES

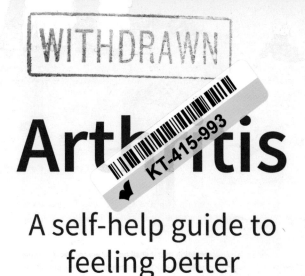

ARTHRITIS: A SELF-HELP GUIDE TO FEELING BETTER

First published in 2010 as *50 Things You Can Do Today to Manage Arthritis*
This revised edition copyright © Wendy Green, 2016

Vie Books is an imprint of Summ

Summersdale Publishers Ltd
46 West Street
Chichester
West Sussex
PO19 1RP
UK

www.summersdale.com

Printed and bound by CPI Group (UK) Ltd, Croydon, CR0 4YY

ISBN: 978-1-84953-806-0

Substantial discounts on bulk quantities of Summersdale books are available to corporations, professional associations and other organisations. For details contact Summersdale Publishers by telephone: +44 (0) 1243 756902, fax: +44 (0) 1243 786300 or email: nicky@summersdale.com.

Disclaimer
Every effort has been made to ensure that the information in this book is accurate and current at the time of publication. The author and the publisher cannot accept responsibility for any misuse or misunderstanding of any information contained herein, or any loss, damage or injury, be it health, financial or otherwise, suffered by any individual or group acting upon or relying on information contained herein. None of the opinions or suggestions in this book is intended to replace medical opinion. If you have concerns about your health, please seek professional advice.

To my husband Gordon, thanks for being so supportive

Acknowledgements

I'd like to thank Susan Oliver, nurse advisor to the National Rheumatoid Arthritis Society, for kindly agreeing to write a foreword. Thanks also to Jennifer Barclay for commissioning this book and to Anna Martin and Sarah Scott for their very helpful editorial input.

Contents

Author's Note

About eight years ago, when I was in my early forties, I began suffering from neck and shoulder pain and stiffness. I ignored it for as long as I could, but eventually, tired of suffering pain on a daily basis, I visited my GP. I was referred to a physiotherapist, who confirmed that I had osteoarthritis in my neck. She showed me how to do gentle exercises to help relieve the pain and advised me against sleeping in my favourite position – on my front with my head twisted to the right or left. Working full-time in a busy college, I found it difficult to fit the exercises into my daily routine and for a while I simply put up with the pain. When the pain got worse after a particularly stressful time at work, I began visiting a chiropractor. I found that manipulation worsened my symptoms at first, but it did eventually bring about some improvement. However, due to the cost and the time involved, I decided this wasn't something I could continue in the long term.

I didn't want to take painkillers or anti-inflammatory drugs on a daily basis, so I began taking fish oil and evening primrose capsules and noticed a slight improvement. I've since learned that working on a computer for hours on end makes the pain worse, so I try to get up and move around every couple of hours or so. Over the past few months, I've found attending a yoga class each week, and swimming whenever I can, extremely beneficial; both the pain and stiffness have improved. I've also recently begun applying capsaicin gel to my neck and shoulders each evening and have found it a great pain reliever. Whilst there is no 'cure' for arthritis, I believe it is possible to manage the condition and lead a full and happy life – it is a case of discovering what works best for you. For many people, lifestyle changes and 'natural' treatments alone will not be enough to control their arthritis symptoms; an integrated approach, combining lifestyle changes with complementary therapies and appropriate medications, is often the most effective.

Wendy Green

Foreword

This book is an excellent resource for anyone who wishes to take some control over their arthritis and to understand whether there is any evidence to support yet another of those well-advertised 'miracle options'. The author balances all the information for you in a quick and easy format that allows you to dip into this book.

As a nurse working in the field of rheumatology, I know how vital it is that people with arthritis get the right information, which includes advice on drug therapies and medical management, at the right time, but also, just as importantly, advice on how to get the best out of managing the condition themselves.

This book contains many of the topics that people with arthritis need to know about, especially in the early days of their arthritis. The information on lifestyle choices, like diet and exercise, and the tone of the writing, which gives information in an upbeat and cheerful way, are aspects of this book that I heartily endorse. There is always something that can be done for arthritis, and this book gives the individual much to focus on.

Susan Oliver,
nurse advisor to the National Rheumatoid Arthritis Society

Introduction

According to the charity Arthritis Care, over nine million people in the UK suffer from arthritis. It is the most common long-term health condition – around one in five adults and 12,000 children are affected. Women are more likely to develop arthritis than men, which suggests a link with female hormones. One in four of all visits to GPs in the UK are in connection with some form of arthritis, and the condition is thought to cost the NHS and social services around five-and-a-half billion pounds each year.

This book mainly focuses on the two commonest forms of arthritis – osteoarthritis and rheumatoid arthritis – and explains how genetic, biological, hormonal, lifestyle and psychological factors can play a part in the disease. It offers practical advice and a holistic approach which, alongside appropriate medical care, will help you manage your symptoms. You'll discover foods and supplements that may be beneficial and learn how to manage stress and relax, and to prevent and ease pain. You'll find information about the best types of exercise for improving mobility and relieving pain and learn about medications and other treatments for arthritis. Practical tips to make everyday living easier and techniques from complementary therapies are also included. At the end of the book you'll find details of helpful products, books and organisations.

Famous arthritis sufferers

- Crime novelist Martina Cole developed rheumatoid arthritis in her late teens. She believes the condition was triggered after she fell from a swing and broke both of her arms at the age of ten. The break in her right arm was the most severe; after it had healed she began to experience pain in her right elbow. A few years later she began to suffer from the symptoms of rheumatoid arthritis – her elbow would throb with pain and her hand would become burning hot. When Martina was 20, a doctor warned her she would be in a wheelchair by the age of 40. She is now 50 and, through sheer determination and a combination of diet, complementary treatments and conventional medicine, Martina has proved the doctor wrong. Although she is by no means 'cured' and she still has painful flare-ups, she has so far avoided severe disability. Her regime includes eating lots of oily fish and taking fish oil supplements, as well as avoiding acidic foods, such as tomatoes and red wine, and taking slow-release ibuprofen tablets. She recently installed a sauna in her home in the hope that the heat would ease the pain.

- The actress Jane Asher, president of Arthritis Care, began suffering from arthritis symptoms at the tender age of seven, though it wasn't until she was older and pregnant that she was diagnosed with ankylosing spondylitis – a form of arthritis that attacks the spine and ribs. She says she has managed to keep her symptoms under control by following an exercise programme and taking anti-inflammatories.

- The explorer Sir Ranulph Fiennes first experienced the pain of arthritis in one hip and both hands when he was in his forties. However, he claims that he has kept his symptoms at bay for over 30 years by taking cider vinegar and honey, as recommended by his mother, Audrey. She began taking the natural remedy, along with molasses and Epsom salt baths, after arthritis in her back left her bedridden. Eighteen months into the regime, her condition began to improve and the pain diminished.

- Hollywood actress Kathleen Turner first developed rheumatoid arthritis at the age of 38. It took her a year to receive the correct diagnosis and she found the illness debilitating. At first, she was given a cocktail of prescription drugs, but she was eventually treated with steroids, which made her look puffy and bloated, giving rise to rumours that she was either an alcoholic or a drug addict. At the time she was neither, but she decided not to reveal that she had arthritis because she feared no one would offer her work if she did. Ironically, seven years later, she discovered that vodka eased the pain and she began using alcohol to help her cope. Eventually, after blacking out in a restaurant, she sought help to give up drinking. She said recently that, thanks to a combination of disease-modifying drugs, swimming and exercising with light weights, her arthritis is now in remission.

Chapter 1

About Arthritis

This chapter gives you an overview of what arthritis is, including the commonest forms of the disease and their symptoms. It also discusses the various factors that may be involved, including age-related degeneration of cartilage, gender, excess weight, joint overuse and injuries, genetics, infections, female hormones, stress, diet and smoking.

❶ Learn about arthritis

Arthritis is a term used to describe joint inflammation. The word comes from the Greek words *arthros*, meaning joint, and *itis*, meaning inflammation.

About synovial joints

A joint is where two bones connect. Most joints are movable joints, otherwise known as synovial joints, because they are lubricated with a liquid called synovial fluid. The purpose of a joint is to enable smooth and flexible movement. The bones are held together by ligaments, whilst tendons attach muscle to bone. A tough, flexible tissue called cartilage, which contains various proteins, including collagen, covers the ends of each bone, to help them glide over each other smoothly and to act as a shock absorber. The joint is encased in a tough, fibrous capsule (called the joint capsule) that protects it and holds it in place. The joint cavity in between the two cartilages is lined with synovial membrane (also known as the synovium), a delicate tissue that releases synovial fluid to provide nutrients and lubrication. Flattened sacs called bursae, which also contain synovial fluid, act like cushions to allow the muscles and tendons to slide over each other without friction, whenever the joint moves. The knees are the biggest joints in the body and support the most weight.

Common types of arthritis and their symptoms

There are over 200 types of arthritis – the two commonest types are osteoarthritis (OA) and rheumatoid arthritis (RA). Whilst both of these conditions can cause similar symptoms, such as pain, stiffness, swelling and limited movement, there are several major differences:

Osteoarthritis (OA)

The result of some form of joint trauma, e.g. overuse, bad posture or excess weight, which leads to loss of cartilage and inflammation.

Only the joints are affected, (usually just one or two, but occasionally more).

Can develop in just one side of the body.

Rheumatoid arthritis (RA) aka Inflammatory arthritis
Caused by the immune system attacking the joints, resulting in inflammation.

Usually symmetrical – affecting the same sites on both sides of the body.

Other parts of the body can also be involved, including the lungs, heart and eyes.

Other, less common forms of the arthritis include lupus, gout, ankylosing spondylitis, psoriatic arthritis and reactive arthritis.

What is osteoarthritis?

Osteoarthritis (OA) is a condition where the joint cartilage thins and roughens. The bone below then tries to repair the damage, but sometimes 'overgrows', leading to new bony outgrowths or 'spurs' on the joints, known as osteophytes. Eventually, as the cartilage wears away, the bones may rub together, causing pain and inflammation. Also, the joint capsule thickens and more synovial fluid may be produced, leading to swelling in the joints. In severe cases the cartilage disappears altogether and the joints become so mishapen that they push the bones out of their normal position, causing deformity.

Unlike many other forms of arthritis, OA affects the joints only and is thought to be largely due to 'wear and tear'. In effect, OA is a process where the body tries to repair damaged joint tissue. In some cases the joint eventually becomes symptom free, but with a different structure. But in some people this process is unsuccessful – perhaps as a result of ongoing or extreme trauma to the joint, or a reduction in the body's ability to heal itself – and the joint damage continues.

Osteoarthritis statistics

8.75 million people in the UK suffer from OA. Around half of people reaching the age of 65 have the condition, with symptoms ranging from mild (especially in the early stages of the condition) to severe; around one in ten sufferers aged 65 and over experience severe disability as a result of OA – especially in one or both hips or knees.

What are the symptoms of osteoarthritis?

The main symptoms are those affecting the joints. They usually occur in the fingers, thumbs, hips, knees, spine (including the neck), ankles and sometimes the shoulders and elbows and include:

Pain
The pain is mainly due to damaged joints and tense muscles. It can come and go, but tends to increase the more the joint is used – hence the pain is often at its worst in the evening – but improves with rest.

Stiffness
The stiffness usually eases after rest, but joint movement may be limited and the joint may 'crunch' or 'creak' as it moves – this is called 'crepitus'.

Swelling
Swelling of the joints might be due to the synovium swelling slightly and producing more synovial fluid, or it may be down to the presence of osteophytes. The knees are especially prone to swelling after exercise.

Loss of balance

Instability, or loss of balance, when moving about. Some OA sufferers say that their joints 'give way'.

Reduced mobility and flexibility

All of these symptoms, depending on their severity, can make you less mobile and less able to carry out everyday tasks. For example, if your hips and knees are affected, you may find walking difficult, and if your fingers and thumbs are affected, you may have problems turning a tap on and off, or opening a jar.

Calcification

This is a fairly common complication of OA. It occurs when calcium deposits form in the cartilage. If these deposits work their way into the synovium, they can cause irritation and hot, painful, swollen joints.

Why do we feel pain?

Pain is the body's way of telling you that something is wrong. Irritation or injury triggers the nerves nearby to release chemicals that in turn stimulate nerve fibres to send messages to the brain, which are interpreted as pain. Pain is often a warning that you need to take action – for example if you touch a hot iron you will automatically respond by removing your hand, to avoid further injury. The pain of arthritis may indicate joint swelling, inflammation or damage. Increased pain might suggest that you have done too much and need to rest, or that you've been sitting in one position for too long and need to get up and move around.

Diagnosis of osteoarthritis

Your GP will probably be able to diagnose OA if you present with these symptoms and signs. Your GP may examine your joints to check for tenderness, swelling and bony growths and may want to see if your movement is restricted. Your GP may also ask if your joints 'creak' or 'crunch' when you move them and may suggest a blood test to rule out other inflammatory forms of arthritis, such as RA. An X-ray may be requested to confirm OA, because it shows changes to the bone caused by cartilage thinning, calcification and bony outgrowths on the joints. However, an X-ray can't predict the level of pain and disability you might experience. Occasionally an MRI (magnetic resonance imaging) scan may be used – this shows the soft tissues such as cartilage, muscles and tendons that don't show up on an X-ray.

What causes osteoarthritis?

There is no single cause of OA, but there are several factors that can raise the risk of developing it.

Age-related degeneration

Although OA can sometimes develop in young people, it more commonly develops from the late forties onwards. This is probably down to changes in the body that tend to develop as the body ages, such as the muscles weakening, weight gain and a reduction in the body's ability to self-heal. However, OA is not an inevitable part of ageing: keeping your weight down, remaining active and avoiding joint strain can all help to keep symptoms at bay.

Gender

Before the age of 45, OA is more common in men. However, among those over 55, women are more likely to be affected, which suggests a link with the menopause; some research suggests that oestrogen protects cartilage from inflammation and this effect is lost after the menopause. Another factor that has been suggested is that women's tendons are more elastic than men's to enable them to give birth; this means that their joints are less stable and more prone to injury. Some experts link it to female anatomy; women's hips are wider than men's to make pregnancy and childbirth easier, which means their knees are not quite as aligned with their hips and this puts more strain on the knee joints. It may also be because women have smaller, weaker bones than men, which are less able to withstand wear and tear.

According to Arthritis Research UK, twice as many women as men develop OA in their hands and four times as many women as men have OA in their knees. Equal numbers of men and women develop OA in their hips.

Obesity

Being overweight puts extra strain on the weight-bearing joints, especially the hips, spine and knees, and not only greatly increases your chances of developing OA, but also makes it worse once it has developed.

Joint overuse or stress

If a joint is overused, or put under stress – for example through bad posture, repetitive use of the finger joints whilst using a keyboard at work, or through participating in a sport – it is more likely to develop OA at some point.

Joint injury

If you injure a joint, for example whilst playing sport, or through an accident, OA may develop in the affected area later on in life.

Other forms of arthritis

Having another form of arthritis, for example RA or gout, increases the risk of developing OA.

Nerve conditions

Nerve conditions such as peripheral neuropathy, which affects the nerves in limbs, may raise the risk of developing OA. Peripheral neuropathy can be caused by other health problems, such as diabetes or alcoholism.

Genetics

Some rare forms of OA that develop in young people and affect the production of collagen (a major component of cartilage) have been linked to particular genes. A form of arthritis known as nodal osteoarthritis, which tends to affect the hands of middle-aged women, has a strong genetic link. However, in general, heredity plays a minor role, compared to the other factors mentioned above.

Heberden's and Bouchard's nodes

Heberden's and Bouchard's nodes are a sign of nodal osteoarthritis. Heberden's nodes are osteophytes on the end joints of fingers, named after the eighteenth-century English physician William Heberden. Bouchard's nodes are osteophytes found on the middle joints of the fingers, named after the nineteenth-century French pathologist Charles-Joseph Bouchard.

What is rheumatoid arthritis?

Rheumatoid arthritis (RA) is a chronic (persistent), destructive inflammatory disease where the immune system attacks the lining of the joints and other parts of the body, including the tendons, ligaments and bones. The disease tends to flare up (relapse), usually for no obvious reason, and then disappear again (remission), sometimes for months, or even years. The affected joints may be damaged during each relapse, gradually increasing disability. This damage can range from mild to severe and usually affects the hands and fingers, making everyday tasks difficult to carry out; around 40 per cent of sufferers are forced to give up work within five years of developing the illness. In a small proportion of cases, the disease progresses continuously and fairly rapidly, leading to severe joint damage and disability.

Rheumatoid arthritis statistics

Around 400,000 people in the UK are thought to suffer from RA. It is three times more common in women than men and, though it can develop at any age, it usually starts after the age of 40. The condition is thought to cost the NHS in England alone around £560 million each year. The total cost to the UK economy each year, including NHS, carer, nursing home, sickness and incapacity benefit expenditure, is thought to be up to £4.8 billion.

What are the symptoms of rheumatoid arthritis?

The main symptoms are usually those affecting the joints. The joints most frequently affected are those in the hands, i.e. the fingers, thumbs and wrists, followed by the feet and ankles. Quite often the knees are implicated. The hips, shoulders, neck and elbows are less commonly involved. The condition often affects the body symmetrically: if the joints in the right hand are affected, those in the left hand are also likely to be. In some sufferers, only one or two joints are involved, whilst others find that several are affected. The symptoms commonly experienced in the joints are:

Pain
This is due to the immune system attacking the synovial membrane that lines the joint (inflammation), damage to the joints, muscle weakness and secondary OA. The pain may continue through the night.

Stiffness
This is usually worse after being inactive, for example first thing in the morning, and usually lasts for more than an hour.

Swelling
The immune response leads to inflammation and swelling in the joints.

Warmth and redness
The inflammation of the joint lining makes the skin over the joint warm, red and swollen.

Joint damage

As the disease progresses, the inflammation damages bone and cartilage and the whole joint can become weakened and deformed.

Loss of joint function

The combination of swelling and joint damage causes a loss of joint function, which makes carrying out everyday tasks, such as getting dressed and performing household chores, difficult.

Other symptoms

Other symptoms of RA that may affect other parts of the body include:

Painless lumps

Also known as nodules, these develop in about a quarter of sufferers – usually on the backs of the hands, the elbows, the forearms and the feet and are generally harmless.

Tendon inflammation

The tissue around the tendons is similar to the synovial membrane around the joints, and can also become inflamed.

Numbness and tingling

Numbness and tingling in the hand – known as carpal tunnel syndrome – can develop when inflammation leads to pressure on the median nerve, the main nerve in the hand.

Tendon rupture

Sometimes the tendons – especially those on the back of the fingers – can rupture as a result of RA.

Inflammation of the blood vessels

RA can cause inflammation of the blood vessels, which can cause problems in any organ, including the heart, but the skin is most often affected. The inflammation can cause bleeding into the skin, which manifests as a rash called purpura, or there may be skin ulcers.

Fatigue

This is likely to be mainly due to the chemicals released during the immune response and is similar to the fatigue you experience when your body is fighting off a flu virus. Also, being in constant pain can wear you down and lead to disturbed sleep.

Low-grade fever

Autoimmune diseases like RA can cause fever – a sign that the immune response is active.

Feeling unwell

During a flare-up you may experience flu-like symptoms and feel generally unwell.

Weight loss

The condition can reduce the appetite, causing weight loss.

Dry eyes

The inflammation can affect the tear glands, causing dry eyes and irritation.

Dry mouth

The salivary glands can also become inflamed, causing a dry mouth.

Anaemia

Anaemia can occur if the bone marrow is affected and fails to produce enough red blood cells. Common symptoms include fatigue, palpitations, shortness of breath and a pale complexion.

Autoimmune disease

The immune system is designed to fight off foreign substances, such as bacteria and viruses, using various specialist white blood cells. In an autoimmune disease like RA, the immune system wrongly identifies healthy tissue in the body as a foreign 'invader' and attacks it. Autoimmune diseases are more common in women than men; female hormones are thought to influence immune activity.

Other conditions associated with RA

RA sufferers have an increased risk of developing other conditions, including heart disease, stroke, joint and other infections, certain cancers, lung diseases, gut problems, and osteoporosis (thinning of the bones):

Heart disease and stroke

RA can affect the heart, causing a build-up of fluid around it. Also, heart disease and stroke are both linked to insufficient physical activity and high blood pressure. People with RA may find it difficult to take exercise and some of the medications used to treat the condition can raise blood pressure.

Joint and other infections

Some of the medications used to treat rheumatoid arthritis suppress the immune system, which leaves sufferers more vulnerable to infections.

Cancer

RA sufferers are twice as likely to suffer from non-Hodgkin lymphoma. This is thought to be because the condition is an autoimmune disease, which means there is increased activity and division within the immune cells, a situation in which cancers of the immune system, i.e. lymphomas, certain types of leukaemia and multiple myeloma (bone marrow cancer), can develop. Sufferers also have a 25 to 50 per cent higher risk of developing lung cancer. This can be linked to rheumatoid lung disease (see below) and the fact that RA sufferers are more likely to have smoked.

Lung diseases

Various lung diseases can occur if the inflammation affects the lungs. Pleural effusion and interstitial lung disease are the two main lung conditions linked to RA. In pleural effusion the lungs and pleura (membrane covering the lungs) become inflamed, leading to a build-up of fluid between the lung and the chest wall. In interstitial lung disease there is swelling and scarring of the air sacs in the lungs. Lung infections can result from taking medications for RA that suppress the immune system.

Osteoporosis

Inflammation can lead to bone loss. Steroid drugs used to treat RA and reduced mobility also raise the risk of developing osteoporosis.

Gut problems

Medications used to treat RA, such as non-steroidal anti-inflammatory drugs (NSAIDs), can irritate the lining of the stomach and cause stomach problems, including diarrhoea.

Diagnosis of rheumatoid arthritis

Rheumatoid arthritis can be hard to diagnose because other types of arthritis can cause similar symptoms. On your first visit, your GP will probably carry out a physical examination to check your joints for swelling and to see how easily they move. Your GP will also want to know about your symptoms. A report on services for people with RA by the National Audit Office in 2009 found that people with RA visit their GP an average of four times before being referred to a specialist. So, to help your GP make the right diagnosis, it's essential that you mention all of your symptoms. If you're worried you might forget some of them, take a record with you. If your GP suspects RA, you may be referred to a specialist for further tests, which are likely to include:

Blood tests

There is no single blood test that can indicate RA. However, there are several tests that can suggest that you may have developed the condition, but they do not definitely confirm it.

Erythrocyte sedimentation rate (ESR)

In an ESR test, a sample of your red blood cells is put into a test tube of liquid. It is then checked to see how quickly the cells fall to the bottom of the tube. If they sink more rapidly than normal, you may have an inflammatory condition such as RA.

C-reactive protein (CRP)

CRP is another test that can detect inflammation in the bloodstream. CRP is produced by your liver and this test investigates how much CRP is present in your blood. A higher level of CRP than usual shows there is inflammation in your body.

Full blood count

A full blood count may be done to check for anaemia. Anaemia is a condition where the blood cannot carry enough oxygen because of a lack of blood cells. Eighty per cent of rheumatoid arthritis sufferers have anaemia. However, anaemia has other causes, such as a lack of iron in your diet, having cancer or being pregnant, so having anaemia does not necessarily mean that you have rheumatoid arthritis.

Rheumatoid factor

This blood test checks whether a specific antibody called 'the rheumatoid factor' is present in your blood. This abnormal antibody is present in 80 per cent of people with RA but it is also found in five per cent of people who don't have RA and it isn't always apparent in the early stages of the disease. As a result, its presence, or absence, does not definitely confirm, or rule out, that you have the condition.

X-rays and magnetic resonance imaging (MRI) scans

X-rays of your joints can help to distinguish between the different types of arthritis. MRI scans use magnetic and radio waves to produce images of your body. MRIs can indicate how much damage has been done to a joint.

What causes rheumatoid arthritis?

It's likely that there is no one single cause of RA – various factors seem to be involved, including genetic, environmental, hormonal, lifestyle and psychological factors.

Genes

Research suggests a genetic link in the development of RA. Several genes that are involved in the immune system are associated with an increased risk of developing the condition. If one identical twin develops RA, the other twin is 20 times more likely to develop the disease than a member of the general population. However, genes are not the 'cause' of RA, they merely predispose a person to the condition – a lot depends on other external factors. In some people, exposure to just one of these other factors may trigger RA, whereas in most people the effects gradually build up until their individual threshold at which RA develops is reached.

Infections

It's thought that infections can trigger RA in a substantial number of cases. It seems likely that when the immune system responds to an infection it doesn't subsequently 'switch off', for some unknown reason. Immunisation, which also stimulates the immune response, has also been linked to the onset of RA in some people.

Hormones

RA is more common in women than in men, which suggests a link between female hormones and its development. The disease rarely starts during pregnancy – in fact it tends to improve. Breastfeeding can sometimes make it worse – possibly because the hormone prolactin, which stimulates milk production, increases inflammation. Women who have never taken the contraceptive pill are around twice as likely to develop RA as those who have. Experts are unclear about whether the contraceptive pill offers long-term protection against RA and there is no evidence that it can improve symptoms in women who already have the disease. Nor is there any evidence that Hormone Replacement Therapy (HRT) has any effect on the development of RA.

Stress

There is evidence to suggest that stress can increase inflammation in the body. Suffering from RA can be stressful – leading to a vicious cycle of physical and psychological symptoms.

Diet

Some nutritionists believe that a poor diet leads to inflammation in the body – possibly triggering RA.

Smoking

The risk of developing RA is much higher in smokers and it is thought that smoking affects the course of the disease. Whilst smoking seems to help to reduce pain and joint tenderness, making it harder for smokers with RA to give up the habit, those who continue to smoke are at greater risk of developing nodules, lung disease and vasculitis (inflammation of the blood vessels). Because more smokers develop RA, there is a higher number of deaths from lung cancer among RA sufferers than among the general population.

Other forms of inflammatory arthritis

There are several other inflammatory forms of arthritis. These include juvenile idiopathic arthritis, lupus, gout, ankylosing spondylitis, psoriatic arthritis and reactive arthritis.

Juvenile idiopathic arthritis

Juvenile idiopathic arthritis, otherwise known as juvenile rheumatoid arthritis or juvenile chronic arthritis, affects around one in a thousand children in the UK. Like RA, the main symptoms are hot, red, swollen and stiff joints. However there are several forms of the disease and each has specific additional symptoms. The three main ones are oligoarticular juvenile idiopathic arthritis, polyarticular juvenile idiopathic arthritis and systemic juvenile idiopathic arthritis:

Oligoarticular juvenile idiopathic arthritis

This mostly affects girls below the age of eight and boys above that age. It involves four or fewer mainly larger joints, such as the ankles, knees or wrists. Boys who develop it over the age of eight may go on to experience stiffness in the lower back and neck. The condition may also cause eye problems. The long-term prognosis is good – most children recover and go on to lead normal lives.

Polyarticular juvenile idiopathic arthritis

This can affect children of either sex at any age, including babies. It affects five or more joints – especially those in the hands and feet. The disease can also attack the neck, jaw and hips. It can quickly spread from one joint to another or it can strike several joints at once and may be accompanied by general ill health, a fever and a rash.

Systemic juvenile idiopathic arthritis

This affects boys and girls equally at any age. Additional symptoms can include a rash, fever and swollen glands, so it is often initially misdiagnosed as an infection. There may also be weight loss, tiredness and fatigue.

There is no cure for juvenile idiopathic arthritis but, as with RA, the symptoms may come and go. Treatment includes regular weight-bearing exercise such as walking, running or aerobics. Swimming is also helpful. Heat or ice treatments may also be beneficial and medications that may help include non-steroidal anti-inflammatory drugs (NSAIDs) such as ibuprofen. In severe cases, steroids or disease-modifying anti-rheumatic drugs (DMARDs) such as methotrexate, may be prescribed. For advice on helping your child to cope with arthritis see Chapter 7 – Living with Arthritis.

Lupus

Lupus is another form of arthritis where the immune system attacks the body. It gets its name from one of its common signs – a butterfly-like rash that was once thought to look like a wolf's bite – lupus is the Latin word for wolf. Around 10,000 people in the UK are thought to suffer from it. Like RA, it affects women far more than men – around 90 per cent of sufferers are women. It tends to strike between the ages of 14 and 50. It can be inherited, so if a member of your family has lupus or some other autoimmune disease, such as rheumatoid arthritis or thyroid problems, you have a higher risk of developing it. Afro-Caribbeans and Asians are more likely to suffer from lupus than other races. The two most common types of lupus are systemic lupus erythematosus (SLE), which can affect any part of the body and can be serious, and discoid lupus erythematosus (DLE), a milder condition that affects the skin and resembles psoriasis.

The main symptoms are depression, fatigue, weakness, skin rashes, joint and tendon pain, swollen glands, headaches, migraine, hair loss, miscarriage, mouth ulcers and reactions to insect bites. These symptoms are often linked to other conditions, such as RA, chronic fatigue syndrome, multiple sclerosis, depression, glandular fever, kidney disorders and Raynaud's disease (which causes numbness, pain and pins and needles) – which means that lupus is sometimes misdiagnosed. Any delay in diagnosis can be serious because lupus can irreversibly damage any of the major organs. Although there is no cure for lupus, if it is diagnosed and treated early it can go into remission, which means there is less risk of complications in the future. About one in five people with lupus also have increased blood clotting which can affect any organ – especially the brain and, during pregnancy, the placenta. This condition, discovered in 1983, is called Hughes syndrome, after one of the scientists that discovered it. It can cause headaches, memory loss, deep vein thrombosis, stroke and miscarriage and can be treated with blood-thinning medication such as aspirin.

Gout

Gout is a form of arthritis that causes swelling and pain in the joints, especially at the base of the big toes, but also in the ankles, knees, wrists, hands or elbows. It affects mainly men of any age and is extremely uncommon in women – though postmenopausal women can occasionally develop it. Every year around 250,000 people with gout go to see their GP. Gout is hereditary, but having a parent with the condition does not mean that you will definitely develop it. It is caused when uric acid crystals build up around the joints and cause inflammation. Uric acid is a waste product in the body that is usually passed out in the urine. However sometimes a person either produces too much uric acid or does not excrete enough of it. Gout triggers include stress, tiredness and illness, joint injury, taking diuretics, eating a lot of protein foods and drinking a lot of alcohol.

The main symptoms of gout are swollen, red, hot and extremely painful joints. There may also be a temperature and tiredness. Attacks can last from one to ten days and the joints usually go back to normal in between flare-ups. Rarely, if the attacks are frequent, there may be lasting damage to the joints. If you believe you have gout, it is essential that you visit your GP, as you may need medication that reduces the level of uric acid in the body. Anti-inflammatory drugs help to ease the pain and inflammation, but aspirin should not be taken as it increases uric acid levels in the body. Managing your weight, following a low-protein diet and cutting back on foods that are high in purines (substances the body breaks down into uric acid) such as kidney, mackerel, herring, sardines, mussels and yeast, will help to reduce the number of flare-ups. Drinking less alcohol may also help. Drinking lots of water helps to prevent uric acid crystals from forming.

Ankylosing spondylitis

Ankylosing spondylitis (AS) is an autoimmune disease that causes chronic (persistent) inflammation. This form of arthritis mainly affects the lower spine and the sacroiliac joints, though other joints and parts of the body, including the upper spine, hips, knees, ankles and shoulders, can also be affected at some stage. The sacroiliac joints are the two large joints that link the base of the spine to the pelvis. The name of the disease derives from the Greek words 'ankylosing', meaning bones joining together across a joint, and 'spondylitis', meaning inflammation of the spine.

AS affects about one in 1,000 people in the UK at some time in their lives; around 200,000 people will visit their doctor with the condition each year. It usually starts between the ages of 15 and 35, although it can also develop in children and older adults. It is up to five times more common in men than in women, which is unusual for an autoimmune disease. There is a strong genetic link, but not everyone who inherits a tendency towards the disease will develop it. The symptoms include early-morning pain and stiffness, weight loss, tiredness and feverishness. Other symptoms can include pain in the heel, eye problems – including pain, blurred vision and iritis (inflammation of the iris) – pain or difficulty in breathing or coughing, and heart problems. These symptoms can flare up and then settle down again for many years.

The condition develops in stages. First of all there is inflammation, where the ligaments or tendons are joined to the vertebrae – the bones that make up the spine. This causes damage to the bone and the formation of scar tissue. The body then responds by growing new bone, which bridges the gaps between the vertebrae, fusing them together and limiting movement in the spine. The same process can take place in the sacroiliac joints, eventually leading to the lower back and pelvis fusing together.

The symptoms of AS can range from mild to severe, though they are usually mild to moderate. About 80 per cent of AS sufferers maintain full independence or have minimal long-term disability and are able to lead normal lives. There is no cure for AS, but it is possible to manage the condition with regular low-impact exercise, such as walking and swimming, and the use of anti-inflammatories and other disease-modifying drugs.

Eye care

If you have AS and develop pain or redness in any part of the eye, see your GP immediately, as leaving it untreated can cause loss of sight.

Psoriatic arthritis

Psoriatic arthritis (PsA) is a type of joint inflammation that affects people with the skin condition psoriasis.

What is psoriasis?

Psoriasis causes itchy, red, raised patches on the skin that have silvery scales and can affect a tiny area of the body, or most of the body. These patches can become sore if they are scratched. The areas most often affected include the elbows, knees and between the buttocks.

Like other forms of arthritis, PsA causes inflammation in and around the joints. The cause is not known. In most cases it manifests after the appearance of psoriasis; often people have psoriasis during their teenage years and PsA develops when they are in their forties. However, in some cases, PsA develops first. The symptoms of PsA resemble those of other forms of arthritis. They include joint pain (elbows, knees, hands, feet, base of spine), morning stiffness, stiff back and neck (spondylitis), swollen finger and toe joints, pitted or thickened nails, and tiredness. Because of its similarities to other types of arthritis, PsA can be hard to diagnose. Rest and relaxation techniques may help to prevent and ease symptoms. Regular exercise can help to maintain mobility. Medications used to relieve PsA include non-steroidal anti-inflammatory drugs (NSAIDs) for the pain and stiffness and anti-rheumatic drugs, injected steroids, and biologics to treat the inflammation. Psoriasis is usually treated with ointments, and where necessary with oral medications such as methotrexate, ciclosporin and retinoids (derived from vitamin A) and ultraviolet light.

Reactive arthritis

Reactive arthritis can develop after having an infection or virus, especially parvovirus ('slapped cheek syndrome'), flu, salmonella or chlamydia, and is the result of antibodies attacking the joints. It affects about five in 100,000 people, is most common in men between the ages of 20 and 40 and it appears to have a genetic link. An attack can last from a few weeks to one year. The first symptoms are usually joint pain and swelling in the knees, ankles or toes and these usually develop three to twelve weeks after the triggering infection. Other symptoms include lower-back pain, genital and urinary tract infections, skin rashes and eye infections, as well as weight loss, diarrhoea, fever, fatigue and mouth ulcers.

Reactive arthritis can be difficult to diagnose, as there is no one conclusive test. Treatment might involve tackling the triggering infection with antibiotics and easing the inflammation with NSAIDs or steroids. Healthy eating, rest and relaxation and gentle exercise to keep the joints mobile can help to aid recovery.

Fibromyalgia

Whilst fibromyalgia is not a form of arthritis, as it doesn't affect the joints, some arthritis sufferers do go on to develop it. Fibromyalgia is the name given to a collection of symptoms, including pain and stiffness in the muscles, ligaments and tendons, that may affect one or more parts of the body, such as the arms, legs, neck and back. The term literally means 'muscle pain'. Other symptoms include sleep disturbances, fatigue, depression and irritability, poor concentration, headaches, irritable bowel and sensitivity to bright lights, noise and temperature. It's thought that the pain of fibromyalgia makes sleep difficult, which in turn leads to fatigue. Women are more likely to suffer from fibromyalgia than men, as are people aged 50 to 70 – though it can sometimes affect children and young people. Triggers are thought to include arthritis, depression, illness, accidents, or other traumatic events, such as bereavement.

The illness sometimes settles down on its own, but it can go on for months or even years. There is no one single cure for fibromyalgia, but there are ways to manage the symptoms. Gentle exercise like walking and swimming can relieve pain, lift fatigue and strengthen the muscles, as well as help the sufferer to sleep better. Stretching exercises, such as yoga, are also recommended as they ease stiffness and improve flexibility. The herb St John's wort may help to relieve the depression and insomnia.

What else could it be?

Other conditions that can be misdiagnosed because their symptoms are similar to those of OA and RA include tendonitis and bursitis.

Tendonitis

Tendonitis is where the tendons and joints become inflamed and it often doesn't improve with painkillers. It often affects the neck, shoulders and wrists. According to Philip Conaghan, Professor of Musculoskeletal Medicine at Leeds University and spokesperson for Arthritis Research UK, this condition is often mistaken for arthritis because it feels the same. He says the condition is usually caused by overuse of the joints and tendons and he recommends muscle-strengthening exercises and better posture to reduce the symptoms.

Bursitis

Bursitis is where the bursae (the sacs inside the joints that contain synovial fluid) become inflamed and swollen, causing agonising pain. It often occurs in the hips, as well as the shoulder, knees, ankles, buttocks, thighs and elbows and can be due to excessive pressure on the joints, through bad posture or repetitive use. If the cause is bad posture, once this is corrected the condition usually disappears. Stress, infection and the inflammation from RA, gout or PsA can also trigger the condition. Treatment usually consists of resting the joint and taking anti-inflammatories, such as ibuprofen.

Four arthritis sufferers' stories

Frances, 66

Frances began suffering from mild OA symptoms at the age of 51. She first visited her GP about one-and-a-half years later, after her symptoms began to worsen. Her GP advised her to lose weight, eat healthily and exercise regularly; he particularly recommended swimming and aqua-fit classes. He also initially suggested taking ibuprofen and then high doses of paracetamol and diclofenac (a non-steroidal anti-inflammatory).

Frances told me that her symptoms are worse when she is stressed – especially when she is emotionally stressed or 'overdoing things'. She has also found that the pain is exacerbated when she is more active than usual – for example, after she has done heavy gardening or housework, or walked further than normal. However, on the other hand, she says her symptoms are also bad first thing in the morning and when she hasn't taken enough exercise. Paracetamol, ibuprofen and diclofenac have helped to relieve her symptoms, as have heat rubs and a hot water bottle. Frances has also found varying degrees of relief from taking glucosamine, chondroitin, methylsulfonylmethane (MSM), fish oils, ginger and probiotics. She is also convinced that her exercise programme has helped; she regularly attends yoga and Pilates classes, swims and does aqua-fit.

Kenneth, 62
Kenneth first experienced aches and pains when he was 46 years old, but didn't visit his GP until the symptoms got worse – around two years later. His GP referred him to a specialist and he was diagnosed with RA. After the diagnosis, his GP recommended keeping active by walking and swimming regularly and avoiding drinking too much tea and coffee. Kenneth recently developed nodules on his hands. He says his symptoms are worse when he overdoes things, but he hasn't noticed a link with any particular food or with feeling stressed. Taking paracetamol, ibuprofen and disease-modifying anti-rheumatic drugs (DMARDs) has helped to control his symptoms.

Susan, 62
Susan visited her GP complaining of a swollen knee when she was 49. She was sent for an X-ray and was told afterwards that

'everything was OK'. Within a year she says she had swollen joints 'all over my body'. She again visited her GP and this time she was referred to a rheumatologist who conducted tests before confirming that she had RA. Susan was initially prescribed steroids to control her symptoms. She has since also been prescribed the DMARD methotrexate as well as rituximab, a newer type of drug known as a biologic (because it mimics the effects of chemicals produced by the immune system).

Susan has taken cod liver oil and found that it helps to reduce her symptoms. Over the years she has noticed that emotional stress makes her symptoms worse, as does too much walking. However, so long as she doesn't overdo it, she has found that going for walks is beneficial. She has recently managed to lose weight and has found that this has greatly improved her ability to get around. She says that when the disease is active it is very painful.

Heather, 60

Heather began suffering from stiffness and pain when she was 56 years old. She visited her GP one year later and was referred to a rheumatologist, who diagnosed RA. Heather says that stiffness, rather than pain, is her main symptom. Following diagnosis, her GP recommended stretching and general exercise. She has noticed that her symptoms are worse when she is stressed by things like 'family problems' and 'not having enough time in the day'. She finds that overdoing it in terms of physical activity can make things worse, and sitting too long makes her stiff. Exercise, especially walking, stretching and using an exercise bike, has proved beneficial. She thinks that fish oils help to relieve her symptoms a little. She has taken diclofenac in the past and found it helped to some degree, but she has recently started taking methotrexate and folic acid and is hopeful that this treatment will prove successful.

Each of these arthritis sufferers has learned through experience what makes their symptoms worse and what makes them better. One important point to emerge is that none of these people was diagnosed with arthritis within the first few months of developing symptoms; for three out of the four this was because, like me, they didn't visit their GP early on.

2 Visit your GP

If you suspect you have arthritis – especially an inflammatory form – it is very important that you visit your GP as soon as you can; it is often hard to distinguish between OA and RA without further tests. Susan Oliver, nurse advisor to the National Rheumatoid Arthritis Society, told me: 'There are many different types of arthritis and, for some of these, the most important thing is to seek medical advice urgently – rapid access to treatment may significantly affect long-term outcomes.' The early use of anti-rheumatic drugs can lower the risk of joint deformity by halting the destructive effects of inflammatory forms of arthritis, as well as reduce the likelihood of suffering from long-term disability, heart disease and stroke. Early diagnosis of OA means that you can take steps to prevent further joint damage, such as regular exercise and managing your weight.

Chapter 2

Medical and Other Treatments

Although this book emphasises the value of self-help, it has already stressed the importance of seeking medical advice as soon as possible if you suspect you have arthritis, so I feel it is useful to discuss medical treatments at this point.

Whilst making lifestyle and dietary changes may help to reduce the frequency and severity of your symptoms, it is highly likely that, at least some of the time, you will still need to take appropriate medications to reduce pain and inflammation and improve joint function. I believe that an integrated approach that combines a healthy, anti-inflammatory diet, exercise, stress management and complementary therapies with appropriate medications is the most effective way to manage the symptoms of OA and RA.

This chapter gives an overview of the over-the-counter and prescription-only medications commonly used for the relief of OA and RA symptoms, including: simple analgesics (painkillers); NSAIDs (non-steroidal anti-inflammatory drugs), which include selective COX-2 inhibitors; steroids; conventional and biologic DMARDs (disease-modifying anti-rheumatic drugs); and newer biologic drugs.

Not everyone will suffer side effects from taking medications and there may be others in addition to those listed, so always read the leaflet that accompanies the medication and discuss any concerns with your pharmacist or GP before using it. You can report a suspected adverse reaction to a drug on the Medicines and Healthcare products Regulatory Agency (MHRA) website (see the Directory at the end of the book). Always inform your GP or pharmacist if you are taking any vitamin, mineral or herbal supplements, as these may interact with medications or reduce their effectiveness.

Practical self-help treatments to relieve pain and stiffness are also included in this chapter, and it ends with a brief overview of the surgical procedures available on the NHS if your quality of life is being severely affected by arthritis pain or if your joints are so damaged you are unable to carry out simple everyday tasks.

Money-saving tip

Ask your pharmacist for generic versions of medications. They are the same drugs, but without the brand name, and can be up to 75 per cent cheaper.

3 Learn about medications for arthritis

Listed below are details of the main medications used to treat arthritis, including what they are, what they are used for, how they work and some of their potential side effects.

Simple analgesics

What they are: Simple analgesics are pain relievers. The over-the-counter drug paracetamol and the prescription-only drug codeine are the two main pain relievers recommended by the National Institute for Health and Clinical Excellence (NICE) for OA and RA.

Good for: Relieving pain.

How they work: Paracetamol blocks the production of hormone-like substances called prostaglandins in the brain and spinal cord, which make nerve endings more sensitive to pain. This means you feel less pain. Codeine blocks pain signals from the nerves to the brain.

Pros: Paracetamol is the cheapest and safest analgesic, as it doesn't irritate the stomach lining and generally has few side effects. Codeine is suitable for severe pain that isn't relieved by paracetamol.

Cons: Analgesics don't reduce inflammation, so they don't relieve stiffness or swelling. Codeine can cause drowsiness, dizziness, nausea and constipation.

Cautions: Paracetamol is toxic to the liver, so overdosing is potentially very dangerous. It's important not to take more than one product containing paracetamol at a time; remember that paracetamol is often included in cold and flu remedies and other preparations. If you are pregnant or breastfeeding, or have liver or kidney problems, let your GP or pharmacist know before taking paracetamol or codeine. If you have breathing, prostate or thyroid problems, or suffer from low blood pressure or epilepsy, let your GP or pharmacist know before using codeine.

Paracetamol dosage guidelines

If you suffer from constant pain, you can take paracetamol throughout the day. The recommended adult dose is one to two 500 mg tablets, up to four times a day (every four to six hours). It is a relatively safe medication and side effects are rare, providing you do not take more than the recommended amount. However, if you find that you need to take painkillers continuously over long periods, it is worth reassessing your lifestyle to determine what is triggering your symptoms and adopting appropriate preventative strategies, such as exercise and relaxation.

Non-steroidal anti-inflammatory drugs (NSAIDs)

What they are: Drugs that reduce inflammation in the body. They include oral NSAIDs, such as aspirin and ibuprofen, and topical NSAIDs (applied to the skin), such as ibuprofen gel.

Good for: Reducing inflammation, pain, swelling and stiffness.

How they work: NSAIDs work by blocking the action of a substance in the body called cyclooxygenase (COX), which is involved in the production of prostaglandins. Some types of prostaglandin are released in response to injury and disease, and cause inflammation, pain and swelling.

Pros: Topical NSAIDs are less likely to produce side effects, as much smaller amounts of the active ingredients reach your bloodstream. A low dose of ibuprofen (200 mg), or topical ibuprofen (gels or creams) are considered the least likely to cause side effects.

Cons: Aspirin and ibuprofen can affect the stomach, because they also reduce the production of beneficial prostaglandins, including those that protect the stomach lining. The longer you use NSAIDs and the bigger the dose, the greater your risk of suffering from side effects. Aspirin, in particular, has to be taken in large doses to reduce inflammation.

Cautions: Don't take NSAIDs if you have had an allergic reaction to one in the past, or if you have or have had a peptic ulcer or severe heart failure. NSAIDs should not be taken alongside antihypertensives (drugs that lower blood pressure), methotrexate (an anti-rheumatoid drug), digoxin (a cardiac stimulant), lithium (a mood stabiliser), warfarin (an anticoagulant), tacrolimus (an anti-rejection drug taken by transplant patients), or selective serotonin reuptake inhibitor (SSRI) antidepressants.

If you have high blood pressure, kidney, liver or heart problems, or have suffered a stroke, speak to your GP or pharmacist before taking an NSAID, as they can make these conditions worse. If you are asthmatic and your condition worsens after taking an NSAID, seek medical advice. The most serious potential side effect is bleeding in the stomach. The risk is higher if you are over the age of 65 or you have suffered from bleeding in the stomach in the past. If you are taking an NSAID and develop indigestion or abdominal pain, or if you vomit blood or pass blood or black, tarry stools, stop taking it immediately and see your GP as soon as possible. To minimise the risk of NSAIDs affecting your stomach, take them with or after food. If you experience any other severe side effects, inform your GP or pharmacist. Other less serious side effects include indigestion, feeling sick, vomiting, diarrhoea, rash, headache, nervousness, dizziness, drowsiness, depression, disturbed sleep and tinnitus (ringing in the ears). These should disappear if you stop taking the medication.

Cyclooxygenase 2 (COX-2) inhibitors

What they are: A newer group of NSAIDs that includes celecoxib, etoricoxib and parecoxib.

Good for: Relieving pain, inflammation, swelling and stiffness.

How they work: They cut the production of inflammatory prostaglandins.

Pros: They don't irritate the stomach lining, because they only reduce production of prostaglandins at the sites of inflammation.

Cons: They slightly raise the risk of heart attack and stroke, because they can increase blood pressure and blood clotting and block the heart-protecting effects of COX-2.

Cautions: COX-2 inhibitors can cause an allergic reaction. Don't take them during pregnancy or breastfeeding, if you have heart disease, atherosclerosis (narrowing of the arteries), kidney problems, a blood clotting defect, peptic ulcers or inflammatory bowel disease.

Note The Department of Health recommends that all people who take steroid tablets and immunosuppressants (see below) should have annual flu and pneumonia vaccinations.

Steroids

What they are: Synthetic versions of the steroids that the body produces – they include cortisone and prednisolone. They are available as ordinary tablets, soluble tablets and injections.

Good for: Dealing with acute symptoms of RA (flare-ups).

How they work: They suppress the immune system.

Pros: They work quickly to reduce inflammation.

Cons: Long-term use can cause serious side effects, including increased risk of infections, osteoporosis, weight gain, diabetes, heart disease, high blood pressure and mood changes. After a while, RA symptoms can reappear despite steroid usage.

Cautions: You shouldn't take ibuprofen whilst taking steroids, as this increases the risk of stomach or duodenal ulcers. Don't stop taking steroids suddenly, as you may get serious withdrawal effects – reduce the dose gradually. Speak to your GP or pharmacist before taking steroids if you have any other health problems or you are pregnant, breastfeeding or trying to conceive.

Conventional disease-modifying anti-rheumatoid drugs (DMARDs)

What they are: A group of drugs used to treat rheumatism that includes methotrexate, azathioprine, ciclosporin, cyclophosphamide, sulfasalazine, hydroxychloroquine, gold by injection (Myocrisin) and leflunomide. Methotrexate is often combined with another DMARD. Folic acid is usually prescribed alongside it to help reduce the risk of side effects.

Good for: Slowing down disease progression and delaying joint damage when used early on in RA.

How they work: They suppress the immune response.

Pros: Various studies suggest that methotrexate is probably the most effective drug for RA.

Cons: DMARDs are slow-acting and can have potentially serious side effects, so you must be monitored whilst taking them. For example, they can affect blood-producing cells, so your white blood cell and platelet levels must be checked regularly.

Cautions: Fairly common minor side effects of methotrexate, hydroxychloroquine and sulfasalazine include rash, tummy upsets and headaches. Methotrexate can also cause increased sensitivity to sunlight and mouth ulcers. Long-term use of hydroxychloroquine can interfere with night vision. Methotrexate and sulfasalazine can affect liver function. Azathioprine can cause blood and bone marrow problems – if you notice any unexplained bruising or bleeding, seek immediate medical advice. It can also raise your risk of infections like chickenpox – if you notice any symptoms, or are exposed to chickenpox or measles while taking azathioprine, seek medical advice immediately. Ciclosporin may cause hair overgrowth, headaches, high cholesterol levels, kidney problems, raised blood pressure and tremors. Drink only small amounts of alcohol when taking methotrexate, as it can increase the risk of liver damage. Don't take methotrexate whilst pregnant or breastfeeding or if you have impaired liver function, an infection or an impaired immune system. Don't take sulfasalazine if you are allergic to aspirin. Don't take hydroxychloroquine if you have retinopathy (damaged retinas).

Biologic DMARDS

Biologic drugs mimic the effects of chemicals produced by the immune system and work more quickly than conventional

DMARDS. Various biologic drugs are used to treat RA, including anti-tumour necrosis factors (anti-TNFs) such as etanercept, adalimumab and infliximab, and newer drugs such as rituximab, abatacept and tocilizumab.

Anti-TNF drugs

What they are: Drugs made from living animal or human proteins.

Good for: Severe active RA that has not responded to DMARDs such as methotrexate.

How they work: They block the effects of the TNF protein, which is produced by white blood cells to fight infections.

Pros: Anti-TNF drugs reduce pain, swelling and stiffness in joints, eyes, muscles and blood vessels and may even repair joint damage.

Cons: They have to be given by injection or an intravenous drip and they can increase your risk of developing infections.

Cautions: Anti-TNFs may not be advised if you have had cancer, tuberculosis or other repeated infections, or if you have impaired kidney or liver function. You should not take anti-TNFs whilst pregnant or breastfeeding.

Newer biologics

What they are: A newer type of drug that includes rituximab, abatacept and tocilizumab.

Good for: Treating the symptoms of severe RA, especially in people who don't respond to anti-TNFs.

How they work: They destroy B-cells (white blood cells involved in the production of antibodies), which prevents the inflammation and immune activity that cause rheumatoid arthritis.

Pros: They can slow the progression of RA.

Cons: Because these drugs affect the immune system, they can make you more prone to infections, especially respiratory infections.

Cautions: You may not be given this type of drug if you get out of breath easily or have low antibody levels. These drugs are not suitable if you are pregnant or breastfeeding, or if you have an infection.

TENS (Transcutaneous Electrical Nerve Stimulation) machines

TENS machines are small, portable battery-operated machines with small electrodes that are taped to the painful area. Low-level electrical impulses stimulate the nerves to release pain-relieving chemicals called endorphins and block pain signals to the brain. The treatment isn't painful, but it may cause a tingling sensation. Many people find that using a TENS machine helps to reduce the number of painkillers they need to take.

Try before you buy

Your GP can refer you to a physiotherapist so that you can try using a TENS machine before considering buying one.

Caution: TENS machines shouldn't be used during pregnancy or if you have a pacemaker, heart problems or epilepsy.

4 Try practical self-help treatments

The following strategies may help to relieve pain:

Try ice or heat

Some people find that placing a cold pack, a towel wrung out in icy cold water, ice cubes or even a bag of frozen peas wrapped in a towel on a hot and swollen or aching joint can reduce swelling and relieve pain. Caution: Don't place a cold pack on your neck, as it could make you faint. Don't use cold packs if you suffer from poor circulation, lupus, Raynaud's disease, Buerger's disease (inflammation and clotting of arteries in the limbs), or peripheral vascular disease (PVD). Speak to your GP before using a cold pack if you have high blood pressure or a heart condition.

Other people prefer to use heat, which boosts the circulation, relaxes tense, tight muscles, and helps to soothe pain. This could be as simple as a soak in a warm bath, or applying a heated pad (gel-filled or electrically heated), hot water bottle or wheat pillow to the painful area. Some people find using a sauna or steam room helpful. For stiff, aching hands, fill a washbasin with warm water, apply a little oil (baby oil or olive oil from the kitchen will do) and massage your hands under water. Some RA sufferers find that an electric blanket helps to relieve morning stiffness. Caution: Don't use a heated pad on a joint or skin that is very inflamed. Don't use a pain-relieving cream that generates heat at the same time as a heated pad, as it may burn your skin. Try both ice and heat, to see which one works best for you.

Note You can buy versatile hot/cold gel-filled packs that can be heated in the microwave, or cooled in the freezer – see Useful Products at the end of the book.

Splint painful joints

Splints can be used to support painful or swollen joints when you are performing tasks, or to help ensure they are supported in the correct position during rest. Resting splints help to reduce pain, stiffness and swelling. Working splints help to both reduce and prevent pain and can help to improve grip strength. They are usually made from a light, synthetic fabric and are held in place with Velcro straps. They are available from pharmacies, rheumatology departments, occupational therapy departments and online (see Directory). Your GP, rheumatologist, occupational therapist or physiotherapist should be able to advise you on the type best suited to your needs.

Other practical ways to relieve pain

Other practical ways to relieve pain include learning to relax (see Chapter 5) and taking regular exercise (see Chapter 6).

Challenging pain

The charity Arthritis Care offers a self-help programme called Challenging Pain, which teaches you skills and techniques to manage chronic pain. See their website for details.

5 Find out about surgery for arthritis

As there are risks attached to surgery, it will probably only be suggested if the joint damage affects your ability to carry out everyday tasks and after you and your GP have explored all other treatments and self-management strategies. The main types of surgery available are joint replacement, hip resurfacing, synovectomy, arthroscopy and fusion.

Joint replacement

Joint replacements are very common and can be total or partial, depending on the degree of joint damage. Hip, knee and shoulder replacements are performed the most often, but smaller joints such as hands, elbows and ankles can also be treated. The operation involves removing all or part of the damaged joint and replacing it with an artificial joint made from plastic, ceramic or metal. Joint replacement is usually carried out on people over 60 years of age, because the younger you are when you have surgery, the more chance there is that you'll need repeat operations.

Hip resurfacing

Hip resurfacing is used for less severe damage. The surface of the joint is replaced with half a metal ball and the socket is lined with metal. As much of the underlying bone as possible is left intact.

Synovectomy

A synovectomy involves removing joint lining that is so inflamed because of RA that the joint is hard to use. It is usually performed using keyhole surgery. It isn't a permanent cure, as the inflammation can return.

Arthroscopy

Arthroscopy usually involves removing damaged cartilage using keyhole surgery and is an alternative to a full joint replacement. It is most often performed on the knees.

Fusion

Fusion involves joining together joints that are painful and difficult to move. After fusion you will no longer be able to move the joint, but it should be less painful, more stable and more able to bear weight. It is most often used in the neck and spine, but can also be performed on smaller joints, such as fingers, wrists, toes and ankles.

Other procedures include removing painful tendon coverings, repairing damaged tendons, removing bone, and releasing trapped nerves to relieve pain.

Chapter 3

Eat to Ease Arthritis

This chapter looks at how the food you eat may be implicated in your arthritis symptoms. Most experts agree that eating a healthy, balanced diet and maintaining a healthy weight are the best ways to keep your joints in good condition. Evidence suggests that eating an anti-inflammatory Mediterranean-type diet is particularly beneficial for arthritis sufferers. The anti-inflammatory diet, its main components and how and why they may be beneficial are discussed here and you will find recipes based on the guidelines in this chapter at the end of the book.

Over the past three decades, several dietary regimes for the treatment of arthritis have been published. Whilst there is no 'hard' evidence that these work, many people who have tried them have reported that they have been helped by them. This chapter examines three of the most popular programmes, one of which was devised by an American doctor called Giraud W. Campbell, another by a British nurse called Margaret Hills and another by the well-known British nutritional therapist Patrick Holford.

Food intolerances may sometimes be involved in arthritis symptoms, so 'exclude and challenge' diets are also explained in this section.

The benefits of an anti-inflammatory diet

Research over several years has consistently shown that a Mediterranean-type diet that is rich in oily fish, olive oil and fresh fruit and vegetables and low in red meat, saturated fats and refined and sugary foods, is anti-inflammatory and therefore beneficial for sufferers of both OA and inflammatory arthritis (RA, juvenile idiopathic arthritis, etc.). However, more recently, scientists have recommended 'the anti-inflammatory diet', which is an expansion of the Mediterranean diet and includes additional foods thought to contain anti-inflammatory nutrients, such as wholegrains, legumes, nuts, seeds and spices.

In a recent review of the existing evidence, Professor Philip Calder, a nutritional immunologist at the University of Southampton, concluded that the omega-3 fatty acids found in oily fish and the compounds found in spices 'damp down' the production of chemicals that trigger inflammation, whilst antioxidants found in fruit and vegetables inhibit the action of free radicals, which destroy healthy cells and worsen inflammation. This type of diet also supplies the vitamins and minerals the body needs to make strong, healthy joints and bones – including vitamin B complex, antioxidant vitamins A, C and E, vitamin D, calcium and magnesium.

The anti-inflammatory diet is filling because of its high fibre content, so it can help you to lose excess weight too. Carrying extra pounds puts additional strain on the joints and even modest weight loss can bring about a reduction in pain, especially in the knees and hips. This is because when you walk, the load on the knee joints is equal to four times your body weight – therefore each pound in weight lost means a four-pound reduction in strain on the knees. Fat cells are also thought to release inflammation-causing chemicals, making the symptoms of both OA and RA worse.

Arthritis Research UK states that while dietary changes alone cannot cure arthritis, there is strong evidence that eating oily fish and plenty of fresh fruit and vegetables can help if you suffer from an inflammatory form, such as RA. The British Dietetic Association also recommends this type of diet for OA.

What is inflammation?

The literal meaning of inflammation is 'set afire'. It is the natural response of the immune system to irritation, infection or injury. The purpose of inflammation is to promote healing by destroying any invading organisms and encouraging the removal of debris from dead bacteria or viruses. Symptoms include redness, heat, swelling and pain. Problems occur when the immune system mistakes normal body tissue for 'the enemy' and attacks it.

Anti-inflammatory fats

The foods we eat contain three types of fat – saturated, polyunsaturated (omega-3 and omega-6) and monounsaturated (omega-9). Some types of saturated fats are thought to cause inflammation, while polyunsaturated and monounsaturated are anti-inflammatory.

Saturated fats are mainly obtained from animal sources, such as red meat, butter and full-fat dairy products, as well as processed foods like sausages, burgers, bacon, biscuits, pies and cakes. However, recent research suggests that a healthy diet can include full-fat dairy products such as whole milk, butter and yogurt, as they may help with weight management by helping you to feel fuller for longer; also the types of saturated fat they contain may even help reduce the risk of diabetes and heart disease. Butter (particularly grass-fed) is also rich in vitamin A. On the other hand, processed meats – especially sausages, bacon and burgers – should be eaten sparingly, because the saturated fats they contain are thought to cause inflammation and are associated with heart disease, atherosclerosis (hardening of the arteries) and breast cancer.

Polyunsaturated fats are found in oily fish, nuts, seeds and vegetable oils. The fats and oils we eat are broken down into fatty acids. Some fatty acids can be produced by the body from other substances, but polyunsaturated fatty acids can't be made in the body and have to be obtained from food – hence they are known as essential fatty acids.

Monounsaturated fats are found in olive oil, rapeseed oil (also known as canola oil) and avocados. Eating certain types of polyunsaturated fats and monounsaturated fats is thought to improve arthritis symptoms.

Essential fatty acids

There are two main types of essential fatty acids: omega-3, found in oily fish, nuts and some plant seed oils; and omega-6, found mainly in plant seed oils such as sunflower oil and corn oil. These two types of fatty acids interact with each other and make anti-inflammatory prostaglandins.

There are two forms of omega-3 fatty acids – long chain and short chain. Long-chain fatty acids include eicosapentaenoic acid (EPA) and docosahexaenoic acid (DHA) and are found in oily fish such as sardines, pilchards, mackerel, herring and salmon. Short-chain fatty acids, such as alpha-linolenic acid (ALA), are found in flaxseed oil, rapeseed oil and walnuts.

Long-chain fatty acids are thought to be the most beneficial for arthritis as, although the body may convert short-chain fatty acids into long-chain fatty acids, it's not known if they have exactly the same effects as long-chain fatty acids that come directly from food. Research consistently shows that the omega-3 polyunsaturated fatty acids found in oily fish and fish oil can be helpful for inflammatory types of arthritis.

It is recommended that we eat oily fish between two and four times a week, not only to help with arthritis and other joint pain, but to also prevent heart disease and promote good physical and mental health. If you dislike oily fish, it may be worth taking a fish oil supplement (see Chapter 4 – Supplementary Benefits). Anyone with gout should avoid eating oily fish, because of its high purine content.

Monounsaturated fats

Monounsaturated (omega-9) fats are found in olives, olive oil, rapeseed oil, groundnut (peanut) oil, nuts and avocados. Olive oil is a major component of the Mediterranean diet and various studies have shown that supplementing the diet with it can help to reduce joint pain, shorten the amount of time sufferers experience stiffness each morning and improve grip strength. Research has also shown that including olive oil in the diet leads to lower levels of C-reactive protein (an indicator of inflammation) in the blood, confirming that olive oil reduces inflammation. In 2005, researchers in Philadelphia claimed that a chemical found in olive oil called oleocanthal was responsible for its anti-inflammatory properties.

6 Use olive oil and rapeseed oil

Recent research at the University of Athens Medical School suggests that including olive oil in the diet protects against the development of RA. Two studies were carried out in Greece involving the completion of a questionnaire by RA sufferers and by control groups who did not have the disease. The studies concluded that people who consumed olive oil regularly had around one-third of the risk of developing RA, compared to those who consumed the least. Both the omega-9 fatty acids and the antioxidants found in olive oil are thought to be responsible for its anti-inflammatory effects.

The researchers noted that vegetables cooked in olive oil also had a protective effect. They also pointed out that, as well as consuming lots of vegetables and olive oil, many Greek people don't eat meat, or meat products, during periods of fasting, which make up around six months of the year for those who strictly observe the Greek Orthodox Church calendar. Extra-virgin olive oil contains more beneficial compounds and has more flavour than ordinary olive oil, because it is unrefined. Rapeseed oil makes a good alternative to olive oil, as it also contains essential fatty acids and anti-inflammatory omega-9 fats, but is lower in saturated fats. It is also cheaper than olive oil and is often simply labelled 'vegetable oil' at the supermarket.

Concerns were raised recently about using olive oil for roasting and frying due to its low smoke point – the temperature at which it starts to burn and smoke. It was thought that when the smoke point was reached the beneficial antioxidants broke down and potentially health-harming aldehydes formed. Aldehydes are harmful substances linked with cancer, heart disease and dementia.

However, in 2015 a study at De Montfort University in Leicester, commissioned by the BBC series *Trust Me, I'm a Doctor*, found that olive oil actually produces fewer aldehydes than polyunsaturated fats such as sunflower and corn oils, due to its high monounsaturated fat content, and is therefore a good choice for frying. Rapeseed oil is also suitable for frying, for the same reason.

An American study has also reported that eating cooked vegetables and olive oil may reduce the risk of developing RA. Try roasting vegetables such as peppers and red onions in olive oil. Add fresh herbs such as rosemary or basil for extra flavour and added health benefits.

Getting the balance right

Achieving the right balance between the two essential fatty acids (omega-3 and omega-6) is important, as too much omega-6 can interfere with the body's ability to break down omega-3 oils, which may lead to inflammation. British people's diets tend to contain too much omega-6: a ratio of omega-3 to omega-6 of around 1:10 instead of 1:3. Therefore, you may find it beneficial to cut down on products containing omega-6 oils, such as sunflower cooking oil and margarine, and use olive oil, rapeseed oil and small amounts of butter instead.

7 Eat a rainbow

The World Health Organization (WHO) recommends eating at least five portions of fruit and vegetables every day to ensure that you obtain the vitamins, minerals and antioxidants your body needs for good health. Antioxidants are believed to help to protect the joints, reducing inflammation by 'mopping up' the chemicals (free radicals) that cause it, and therefore potentially helping to prevent arthritis. Recent research suggests that people who eat plenty of fresh fruit and vegetables, especially those containing vitamin C, have a reduced risk of developing inflammatory arthritis. In order to ensure that you consume a wide range of nutrients, it's important to 'eat a rainbow' – in other words, select fruit and vegetables across the colour spectrum, especially those with bright hues such as apples, avocados, blueberries, beetroot, broccoli, cherries, grapes, peppers, raspberries, spinach and sweet potatoes, as these are thought to contain the highest concentrations of beneficial substances.

Fruit and vegetables also provide both insoluble and soluble fibre, helping you to feel full for longer, which is useful if you need to lose weight in order to relieve the strain on your joints.

Try drinking cherry juice for gout

Research at the University of California suggests that Montmorency cherries can help to lower uric acid levels and relieve joint inflammation and pain. You can buy Montmorency cherry juice at most supermarkets (see the Useful Products section).

8 Eat less meat

As well as the previously mentioned research conducted in Athens, other studies suggest that eating less red meat reduces the risk of developing RA. A study commissioned by Arthritis Research UK reported that people who ate red meat every day had twice the risk of developing RA compared to those who ate it less often. The scientists, who evaluated the eating habits of 25,000 people, thought that it might be the collagen in meat that triggers the immune response in some people. Another possible explanation is that meat's high iron content is to blame – it has been suggested that too much iron in your diet may accumulate in the joints and damage them. Try substituting meat dishes for fish-based or vegetarian meals at least twice a week.

9 Snack on nuts and seeds

Vitamin E is an effective antioxidant and some research suggests that people who have high intakes of it are less likely to develop OA or RA than people whose intake of it is low. Nuts (especially almonds) and seeds (especially sunflower) are rich in vitamin E. Other sources include sweet potatoes, avocado and spinach. Nuts and seeds are also a good source of selenium, which is a trace element that is used to make antioxidant enzymes. Research has shown that a lack of selenium may be linked to an increased risk of developing both OA and RA and an increase in the severity of OA. Brazil nuts, macadamia nuts and sunflower seeds are particularly rich in selenium. Other sources include seafood, cereals and meat.

10 Spice up your cooking

According to Professor Christopher Cannon from Harvard Medical School, co-author of *The Complete Idiot's Guide to the Anti-Inflammation Diet*, garlic and spices, especially turmeric, ginger and cumin, may ease the pain and inflammation associated with arthritis. Chillis are also believed to be anti-inflammatory.

- Garlic contains sulphur compounds that are believed to have anti-inflammatory properties.

- Turmeric gets its colour from curcumin, a bright yellow pigment that is thought to have anti-inflammatory properties. It is believed to work by blocking the action of a protein that binds to genes and promotes the release of inflammatory chemicals.

- Ginger has traditionally been used in Ayurvedic (native to the Indian subcontinent), Chinese and Japanese medicine to reduce inflammation and relieve joint problems. An uncontrolled Danish study in 1992 suggested that adding about a teaspoon of fresh ginger root or powdered ginger to food helps to relieve OA and RA symptoms in some people.

- Cumin is the dried seed of the herb *Cuminum cyminum*, from the parsley family. It contains thymoquinone, a powerful antioxidant that appears to reduce inflammation.

- Chillis contain capsaicin, which is thought to be anti-inflammatory and to stimulate the release of endorphins – brain chemicals that have a pain-relieving effect.

Herbal helper

Basil contains a volatile oil called eugenol, which is believed to have anti-inflammatory properties similar to those found in aspirin – hence it may be beneficial to arthritis sufferers. Try adding torn basil leaves to pastas and salads.

11 Eat calcium-rich foods

People with RA, OA and other forms of arthritis including ankylosing spondylitis, systemic lupus erythematosus and polyarticular juvenile idiopathic arthritis have an increased risk of developing osteoporosis (brittle bones). This can be due to the disease itself or the effects it has on mobility – bones need regular weight-bearing exercise to remain strong. Also, the steroids often used to treat arthritis can lead to osteoporosis when taken over a long period of time. Eating calcium-rich foods helps to keep your bones strong and healthy and reduce the risk of developing osteoporosis. Women are more likely to suffer from osteoporosis after the menopause, when they lose the bone-protecting effects of oestrogen. Nutritionists recommend a daily intake of 1,000 mg, increasing to 1,500 mg for people aged over 60.

The richest sources of calcium are dairy foods such as milk, hard cheese and yogurt. One pint of whole milk, one 125 g pot of yogurt and 30 g hard cheese would supply around 1,100 mg of calcium. Tinned sardines are also a good source, if you eat the bones. Good non-animal calcium providers include almonds, seeds, tofu, soya, seaweed, figs, dates, dried apricots,

Brazil nuts, purple broccoli, watercress, leeks, parsnips, lentils, beans and green leafy vegetables such as kale.

To increase your absorption of the calcium they contain, sprinkle leafy green vegetables with a little ordinary vinegar. Drinking a tablespoon of cider vinegar in warm water, sweetened with honey if desired, once or twice a day is also recommended for promoting calcium absorption.

'Good' bacteria – probiotics such as lactobacillus – also seem to improve calcium absorption. Various probiotic foods are available, such as natural live bio-yogurt, which is also rich in calcium, and drinks like Yakult and Actimel.

12 Boost your vitamin D intake

Vitamin D is needed to help the body absorb calcium, and some research suggests that all types of arthritis progress more quickly in sufferers whose vitamin D intake is low.

The body produces vitamin D following exposure to sunlight, which means you can become deficient in it during the winter, so it's important to obtain sufficient amounts from your diet. Margarines, cereals and powdered milk are generally fortified with vitamin D. Other sources include eggs, oily fish and liver. The recommended daily allowance is between 10 and 15 micrograms, or 400–600 international units (IU): vitamin D is only needed in very small amounts, therefore it is usually measured in micrograms or IU.

Boost your intake of other bone-strengthening minerals
Magnesium is also involved in converting vitamin D to the active form needed to ensure calcium absorption, thus helping maintain bone density. And, according to the Health Supplements

Information Service (HSIS – see Directory), magnesium deficiency can lead to joint pain and muscular tension. Nuts, seeds, wholegrains and leafy green vegetables are good sources. Around 60 per cent of the magnesium in your body is stored in your bones.

Zinc stimulates bone formation. Meat, wholegrains, dairy foods, nuts and seeds are good sources.

Epsom salt soak

Boost your magnesium levels and ease aching muscles and joints by taking a long soak in a warm bath containing magnesium-rich Epsom salts. Simply add one to two cups of Epsom salts to the bath as it fills. According to researchers at the University of Birmingham, the greater your deficiency, the more magnesium your body will absorb.

13 Get more iron

Anaemia – the condition attributed to iron deficiency – can be one of the symptoms of RA, so it is important that you regularly top up your iron intake. Good sources of iron include salmon, sardines, tuna, eggs, liver, meat, poultry, dark green leafy vegetables, including spinach, watercress and kale, fortified breakfast cereals, wholemeal bread, nuts, and dried fruits such as prunes and apricots. Vitamin C boosts iron absorption, so try to have vegetables, fruit or fruit juice with your meals. Drinking tea with or after meals can reduce the amount of iron your body absorbs.

> ## Iron supplementation
>
> Don't take an iron supplement without speaking to your GP first, as some researchers believe that too much iron may damage the joints.

14 Treat yourself

An anti-inflammatory diet can also include treats like plain chocolate and wine.

Plain chocolate

Plain chocolate is rich in flavanols, which are antioxidant. For the maximum benefits, go for chocolate containing a minimum of 70 per cent cocoa. However, even dark chocolate can be high in fat and sugar, so try to limit your intake to no more than 25 to 50 g daily.

Wine

Drinking wine in moderation (no more than two 125 ml glasses daily) may be beneficial for arthritis sufferers. Both red wine and white wine contain anti-inflammatory substances. Polyphenols are thought to be the beneficial ingredient in red wine and, according to researchers at the universities of Milan and Pisa, the chemicals tyrosol and caffeic acid found in white wine may prevent inflammatory conditions like RA.

Drink plenty of fluids

The daily consumption of two to three litres of fluids, such as water, unsweetened fruit juices, weak tea and herbal teas, keeps the body hydrated and helps to ensure a steady supply of nutrients to the joints.

15 Learn about anti-arthritis diets

Some experts believe that a poor diet and certain foods can cause both OA and RA symptoms, and advocate anti-arthritis eating plans. The most well-known of these include the special regimes devised by Giraud W. Campbell, Margaret Hills and Patrick Holford. If you decide to follow any of these regimes in the long term it may be advisable to discuss it with your GP or a dietician first, to make sure your diet is balanced.

Dr Giraud W. Campbell's seven-day programme

About 45 years ago, an American doctor called Giraud W. Campbell began treating his patients who had arthritis with a dietary programme that involved avoiding processed foods, bread and other flour products, alcohol and caffeine, and focusing on a healthy diet consisting of fruit, vegetables, fish and dairy foods. He outlined the principles of the diet in his book *A Doctor's Home Cure for Arthritis: The bestselling proven self-treatment plan* (see Helpful Reading). Many people claim to have been helped by this eating plan, including the well-known cook Marguerite Patten.

Dr Campbell believed that all types of arthritis are due to eating a poor diet that is lacking in vital vitamins and minerals and high in additives. His approach is an elimination diet that involves detoxing the body and then introducing wholesome foods gradually and noticing what effect they have on your symptoms. His seven-day programme involves fasting on the first day and then eating lots of fresh, raw fruit (except citrus fruit) and vegetables and lightly cooked liver on the second day. By day three you can include unpasteurised cow's or goat's milk and fish, preferably fresh.

Over the next few days you can add various meats, including beef, lamb, turkey and free-range chicken, one at a time. If symptoms such as stiffness return after eating a particular meat, you should exclude it and then try reintroducing it a week later. Dr Campbell suggested that the stiffness is not likely to return. He said that you should observe your reactions to each new food that you introduce and, if your joint pain returns after eating a particular food, you should add it to your list of culprits and avoid eating it in future.

He also recommended taking cod liver oil and brewer's yeast supplements. He advised permanently avoiding sugary foods such as jams, jellies and sweets, and processed foods such as custard powder and prepared mixes. Perhaps more controversially, Dr Campbell 'banned' all flour products, including those made from soy flour, rye flour, etc., such as bread, cakes, biscuits, noodles and pasta. His diet also excludes tea, coffee, cola and alcohol.

Margaret Hills' drug-free approach

Margaret Hills was a nurse who developed an acid-free dietary approach to arthritis after she developed first RA and then

OA. Hills was 21 and undertaking nurse training when she was diagnosed with RA. She spent the next five months in hospital before being sent home to convalesce. Because her heart had been badly affected by the disease, she was advised to give up nursing and avoid the activities she loved – dancing and cycling.

However, she decided that she wanted to enjoy life, so she ignored the advice and resumed the activities she enjoyed. She soon lost the excess weight she had gained whilst in hospital and, despite also having developed OA, she was allowed to resume her nursing training. She completed her training and married, but continued to suffer from the pain of OA. After 16 years and six children, she suffered another RA attack, which left her crippled. The only treatment available to her, apart from aspirin, was a new 'wonder drug' that her doctor deemed to be unsafe, so she began to research 'natural cures' and went on to develop her own treatment.

From her research, Hills concluded that both OA and RA were caused by an excess of uric acid in the body, caused by a poor diet. Her treatment aimed to remove excess uric acid from her body and provide nutrients to help in the burning up of the acids, as well as preventing any further build-up. It included taking one dessert spoon of cider vinegar and one teaspoon of honey in water three times a day and one teaspoon of black molasses three times daily. She also took vitamin, mineral and protein supplements every day and did regular, gentle exercise. Three times a week she took a bath containing three cups of Epsom salts.

In addition, she followed a healthy, 'acid-free' diet that was low in salt and animal fats and excluded alcohol, citrus fruits, tomatoes, processed meats (such as ham, bacon and sausages) and refined foods like white sugar, white bread, cakes and biscuits. Instead, she based her diet on wholegrains, fish, cottage cheese, lamb (including the liver and heart), rabbit, poultry, fresh vegetables and non-citrus fruits. 'Allowed' drinks included apple juice, weak tea, decaffeinated coffee and the occasional Guinness. She also consciously avoided stress as much as possible.

In her book, *Treating Arthritis: The Drug-Free Way* (see Helpful Reading), Hills reported that, within 12 months, the treatment had rid her of 'all signs of arthritis' and that she remained pain free. In 1982, she opened a private clinic in Kenilworth, Warwickshire, so that she could treat arthritis sufferers using her holistic methods. The clinic is still running today; further details can be found in the Directory.

Patrick Holford's anti-arthritis diet

The nutritional therapist Patrick Holford links arthritis to poor diet, food intolerances, an overgrowth of 'bad' bacteria in the gut, increased gut permeability (where undigested food passes through the gut wall into the bloodstream, triggering inflammation), and an overload of toxins. His approach involves reducing your intake of toxins, increasing your intake of fruit and vegetables and avoiding meat and dairy foods, as well as foods to which you are intolerant. He also recommends taking supplements that support healthy liver function, such as milk thistle, artichoke and dandelion root.

Holford believes that, to combat arthritis, it is essential to maintain steady blood sugar levels. He advocates a low-GI (glycaemic index) diet that focuses on foods that release glucose slowly to help achieve this. The most beneficial low-GI foods, according to Holford, include rye bread, beans, peas, lentils, wholegrains, porridge and oatcakes. He also suggests increasing your intake of essential fats by eating fish, nuts and seeds and their oils, and including herbs and spices such as rosemary, parsley, tarragon, thyme, cinnamon, ginger and garlic in your daily diet.

Discussion

Whilst each of these eating plans differ to some degree – for example, Dr Campbell's and Margaret Hills' regimes include meat and dairy foods, whilst Patrick Holford's doesn't – they all promote the message that one of the best ways to combat arthritis is to eat a wholesome diet and avoid processed foods. Although some aspects of these eating plans remain controversial and unproven, for example the idea that cider vinegar benefits arthritis, or that everyone with arthritis should avoid starches, tomatoes and citrus fruits, they all include many of the current anti-inflammatory dietary recommendations. Therefore, it may be worth considering adopting one of these regimes, even just for a few weeks, to see whether your symptoms improve.

16 Be aware of food sensitivity

If you think you might be allergic or intolerant to certain foods, try excluding them from your diet for one month and see whether your arthritis symptoms improve. Then reintroduce the food and note whether your symptoms flare up again. If the culprit is from a major food group, or if you think you might be sensitive to several foods, it is advisable to ask your GP to refer you to a dietician, otherwise you might run the risk of developing a nutritional deficiency. If you take NSAIDs, be aware that they can increase the permeability of the gut, making it 'leaky'. This means it allows bigger particles of food to pass through than normal, causing food sensitivity. So, if you are able to reduce the amount of NSAIDs you take, you may find that you become less sensitive to different foods.

Foods that have been linked with joint pain in arthritis sufferers include wheat, corn, rye, sugar, caffeine, yeast, malt, dairy products, citrus fruits and foods from the nightshade family – such as tomatoes, potatoes, aubergines and sweet peppers. However, the idea that an elimination diet can help all types of arthritis is not supported by Arthritis Research UK or by Arthritis Care. Both organisations say that an elimination diet, under medical supervision, can help relieve symptoms in some RA sufferers, but argue that there is no evidence that such a diet can help OA sufferers.

Arthritis sufferers' experiences with food

Fenella Barton's story

Violinist Fenella Barton developed RA in her forties, following a stressful relationship break-up. When she was feeling especially low, she began to experience pains in her arms and feet and struggled to complete everyday tasks. Within months she was finding it difficult to get out of bed in the morning and couldn't even summon the strength to squeeze a tube of toothpaste. Believing that she might be suffering from a food allergy, Fenella tried cutting out wheat, then dairy and then acidic foods, but her condition didn't improve. She visited several physiotherapists, some of whom told her she might have arthritis, but she ignored their warnings. As her condition worsened and her muscles wasted, she lost weight and often felt cold.

Over a year later, she discussed her symptoms with a friend who persuaded her to visit her GP. Eventually, following a blood test, she was diagnosed with RA. She was initially prescribed steroids and methotrexate and described the effects as 'like being unfrozen'. However, concerned about the side effects of long-term use of methotrexate, she decided to visit a homeopath. She was advised to follow a low-sugar diet, eat lots of organic vegetables and take 3 g (half a teaspoon) of fish oil each day. When she eventually came off the drugs, some of the aches and pains came back. However, she said recently that she has been symptom-free for over a year but she has been warned that, although the RA was currently inactive, it could flare up again in the future.

Marguerite Patten's story

The well-known cook and food writer Marguerite Patten suffered from severe arthritis and she tried various therapies to control her symptoms, including acupuncture and chiropractic treatments, without success before stumbling upon Dr Giraud W. Campbell's book. She realised that, although the diet appeared strict, it contained many of the foods she enjoyed eating, so she decided to give it a try. She reported a dramatic improvement in her symptoms within weeks and was so enthused by the diet and its beneficial effects that she decided to team up with her nutritionist friend Dr Jeannette Ewin to write a book entitled *Eat to Beat Arthritis: Over 60 recipes and a self-treatment plan to transform your life* (see Helpful Reading). She says that nowadays she doesn't stick to the diet quite as stringently, but that she almost completely avoids tea, coffee and wine and limits her intake of orange juice and wheat to keep her symptoms at bay. If her arthritis pain returns, she follows Dr Campbell's strict diet for a few days.

The anti-arthritis diet

Here is a brief summary of the dietary advice in this chapter:

- Eat oily fish at least twice a week (except if you have gout).
- Use olive, rapeseed, flaxseed or walnut oil for cooking and on salads.
- Avoid eating processed meats and shop-bought baked goods.
- Eat lots of different, brightly coloured fresh fruit and vegetables.
- Cut down on red meat and refined and sugary foods.
- Eat wholegrain foods such as brown rice and wholemeal bread.
- Snack on nuts and seeds.
- Eat legumes (beans, lentils and pulses).
- Use spices such as garlic, turmeric, cumin, ginger and chilli in your cooking.
- Eat foods rich in calcium, vitamin D, magnesium, zinc and iron.
- Drink plenty of fluids.
- If you suspect a food intolerance, try an 'exclude and challenge' diet.

Chapter 4

Supplementary Benefits

Many people concerned about the side effects of the anti-inflammatory painkillers and other medications commonly prescribed for arthritis prefer to treat their symptoms with supplements containing herbs or nutrients that are believed to be beneficial. This chapter gives an overview of many of the supplements commonly recommended for OA, RA and fibro-myalgia and discusses the evidence regarding their effectiveness. It's important to remember that, just because a supplement contains natural substances, it doesn't mean that it's harmless – many plants are poisonous to humans. Also, current legislation means that the content and quality of supplements cannot always be guaranteed. These issues are covered in this chapter.

How effective are supplements for arthritis?

Numerous supplements have been recommended for arthritis; however, according to the second edition of the report entitled 'Complementary and alternative medicines for the treatment of rheumatoid arthritis, osteoarthritis and fibromyalgia', published by Arthritis Research UK in 2012, only 31 have been tested using random controlled trials (RCTs). This doesn't necessarily mean that other supplements are ineffective, but it does mean that reliable research into their effectiveness has not yet been done. RCTs are viewed as the most reliable type of trial because they randomly place participants in either a treatment group or a control group. The treatment group receives the treatment under scrutiny, whilst the control group may receive a placebo or a different treatment for comparison purposes. RCTs can be single-blind, where the participants don't know which treatment they are receiving, or double-blind, where neither the participants nor the researchers know who is receiving which treatment. Of the 31 supplements tested using RCTs, Arthritis Research UK concluded that only 12 had promising or consistent evidence regarding their effectiveness in treating arthritis.

How will I know a supplement is safe?

It's important to remember that just because something is described as natural, it doesn't automatically mean it's safe – like medications, herbs can have side effects, sometimes serious, which can interact with prescription drugs. Also, if you're not careful, you could buy a product that doesn't contain the ingredients it's supposed to, which at the very least will mean you've wasted your money. Worse still, the product might contain other undisclosed and potentially dangerous ingredients. Fortunately, legislation introduced in 2011 has made it easier to check the safety and quality of the product you're buying.

Herbal products are most often sold as either traditional herbal registration (THR) remedies or herbal food supplements. THR products are regulated and monitored by the government organisation known as the Medicines and Healthcare products Regulatory Agency. If a product has a THR stamp it means the MHRA is satisfied that it meets quality standards and has appropriate labelling and a product information leaflet. It also indicates that the herb has been used in traditional remedies for over 30 years. All THR products have a nine-digit registration number starting with the letters THR on the container or packaging.

Also, a few herbal medicines in the UK have a product licence. Licensed herbal medicines, like any other medicine, are required to demonstrate safety, quality and effectiveness, and to provide guidelines on safe use, so only herbal medicines with medicinal claims supported by acceptable clinical data are given product licences. They can be identified by a nine-digit number, prefixed by the letters PL.

The MHRA provides a full list of herbal products currently registered under the Traditional Herbal Medicines Registration Scheme, along with information sheets on their safe use. Details can be found in the Directory at the end of this book.

Herbal food supplements, on the other hand, come under the remit of the Food Standards Agency (FSA), and the Chartered Trading Standards Institute at local authority level, and are not under the same legal and manufacturing scrutiny. This means there is no guarantee of their content or quality. In 2015 the School of Pharmacy at University College London tested over 70 of the herbal remedies most often bought from the high street or online and worryingly found that, while most contained high amounts of the main ingredient, up to a third had very little or none at all. So it is probably best to choose THR remedies or, if a product isn't registered, check that it is from a reputable UK company.

Chinese herbal medicine and your safety

Traditional Chinese herbal medicines are currently unregulated; this has led to concerns regarding the quality and safety of some products. For example, there is some evidence that Thunder God Vine can reduce the symptoms of RA, but it can also cause several unpleasant side effects and it is poisonous if not extracted properly. I feel it is advisable not to use Chinese herbal products unless they have been approved by the MHRA.

The effectiveness score and safety ratings of the 2012 Arthritis Research UK report

This report gave each supplement a score of one to five, according to the strength of the evidence that a compound improved pain, movement or general well-being:

1 = no evidence, or overwhelming evidence of ineffectiveness
2 = only a little evidence
3 = promising, though mixed evidence
4 = some consistent evidence from more than one study
5 = consistent evidence across several studies

Where there was sufficient information regarding the safety of supplements, the report gave the following 'traffic light' ratings:

Green: Minor, infrequent adverse effects.
Amber: Common minor or more serious side effects.
Red: Serious side effects.

The report warned that compounds that are safe when taken as recommended may cause serious adverse effects if higher doses are taken.

To decide whether it is worth continuing to take a supplement, review the benefits it has on your symptoms. Evaluate your level of pain and stiffness on a scale of zero to ten before you start taking the supplement, and then repeat after three months of use.

17 **Benefit from supplements**

Below are some of the supplements commonly recommended for arthritis. To help you select the supplements with the most reliable evidence and best safety record to support their use, the effectiveness and safety ratings of the 2012 Arthritis Research UK report are included. Wherever possible, related products are listed in the Useful Products section at the end of the book.

Borage seed oil

What it is: Also known as starflower oil, borage seed oil is derived from the seeds of the Mediterranean herb borage. Borage seed oil can be bought as oil or in capsule form.

Beneficial effects: It reduces the joint inflammation of RA.

How it works: Contains high levels of the omega-6 essential fatty acids linolenic acid (LA) and gamma-linolenic acid (GLA), both of which have anti-inflammatory properties. LA is converted into GLA in the body, which is thought to reduce inflammation in the body in two ways: it is used to produce prostaglandins (hormone-like substances) that regulate the immune system and it may also dampen inflammation by acting on certain inflammatory cells.

Evidence of effectiveness: In one RCT, 37 participants were given either borage seed oil supplying 1.4 g of GLA or a placebo of cotton seed oil, which they were asked to take daily, alongside their usual treatment, for 24 weeks. Those who took the borage seed oil reported fewer swollen joints and less joint tenderness and morning stiffness, whilst the placebo group saw no change in their symptoms. In another RCT, 56 RA sufferers were randomly given either borage seed oil capsules supplying 2.8 g of GLA or sunflower seed oil capsules. At the end of the trial, 64 per cent of those using the borage seed oil capsules experienced an improvement in joint tenderness and morning stiffness, compared to 21 per cent taking the placebo.

Effectiveness score: 3 (for RA)

Safety: In both RCTs the side effects reported were mild and included burping, wind and diarrhoea.

Safety rating: Green

Capsaicin gel

What it is: Capsaicin is extracted from chilli peppers.

Beneficial effects: It eases the pain associated with OA.

How it works: It reduces the levels of a protein called substance P, which is involved in the transmission of pain signals from the nerve endings to the brain and in inflammation of the joints.

Evidence of effectiveness: In 1994, an analysis of the combined results of three RCTs showed that capsaicin was four times as effective as a placebo at relieving joint tenderness and pain. A six-week RCT in 2000 involved 200 OA sufferers using either a 0.25 per cent capsaicin cream, a placebo cream, a glyceryl trinitrate cream, or a capsaicin and glyceryl trinitrate combined cream. At the end of the trial, all of those who had used a cream with active ingredients, rather than the placebo, had less joint pain and needed fewer painkillers. Those using the cream containing both capsaicin and glyceryl trinitrate reported the greatest improvements. A third RCT looked at the effects of capsaicin gel on fibromyalgia. Forty-five participants were given either 0.25 per cent capsaicin gel or a placebo gel to apply to painful areas four times per day. After a month, those using the capsaicin cream had less tenderness and had much better grip strength than those using the placebo. Capsaicin gel had the highest effectiveness score in the Arthritis Research UK report. It is available on prescription in the UK as a gel or a cream.

Effectiveness score: 5 for OA and 2 for fibromyalgia

Safety: Capsaicin is an irritant, so keep the gel away from your eyes, nose and mouth and open wounds. Always wash your hands thoroughly after applying.

Safety rating: Green

Chondroitin sulphate

What it is: Chondroitin sulphate is a complex sugar and a major component of cartilage, and supplements of it are usually derived from cow, pig, shark or bird cartilage. This supplement comes in capsule form and is often combined with glucosamine sulphate.

Beneficial effects: It prevents and repairs damage to cartilage that is caused by OA.

How it works: It is believed to suppress the action of enzymes and other substances that break down joint collagen and also helps cartilage to retain water, making it more elastic and resilient.

Evidence of effectiveness: In 2009, researchers in Barcelona reported that chondroitin sulphate, either on its own or with glucosamine sulphate, relieved the inflammation and swelling caused by OA in the knee more quickly than paracetamol.

The trials they had conducted involved between 46 and 631 participants and lasted from three months to two-and-a-half years. Sixteen of these trials compared the benefits of chondroitin sulphate with those of a placebo and five trials looked at its ability to reduce narrowing of the joint space, and found that it had only a small effect on that. Twelve trials found that chondroitin sulphate was significantly better than a placebo in relieving pain and reducing the need for painkillers; however, the results of four trials suggested that chondroitin sulphate was no more effective than a placebo. However, in 2010 a review of 22 RCTs investigating the effectiveness of chondroitin sulphate for OA in the hip and knee concluded that chondroitin (on its own or with glucosamine) didn't reduce joint pain to any clinically meaningful extent, or change any clinical aspects of the joint.

Effectiveness score: 2 (for OA)

Safety: Occasional side effects include stomach upset, headache, wind, diarrhoea and skin rash. If you take any medications that thin the blood (such as warfarin) consult your GP before taking chondroitin sulphate, as it may increase their effects.

Safety rating: Green

Devil's claw

What it is: Devil's claw is a plant native to Southern African deserts, where extracts from the plant's roots have long been used to treat arthritis.

Beneficial effects: It relieves the pain associated with OA.

How it works: The active ingredients are thought to be glycosides, especially one called harpagoside, which block inflammatory mechanisms. However, some studies suggest that other plant constituents may be involved.

Evidence of effectiveness: In 2006, a review at the University of Southampton of 14 studies into the effectiveness of devil's claw as a treatment for OA concluded that, despite some of the studies being of poor quality, results from the higher-quality studies suggested it relieved pain. One of the higher-quality studies found that two groups of OA sufferers noted similar improvements in their symptoms after one group was randomly given devil's claw and the other diacerein (an OA drug). However, the group using devil's claw experienced fewer side effects. The Arthritis Research UK report concluded that devil's claw is as effective as conventional OA medications.

Effectiveness score: 3 (for OA)

Safety: Serious side effects are uncommon, but can include an increased heart rate; if you suffer from heart problems, blood pressure problems or diabetes you should speak to your GP before using devil's claw. Other less severe side effects include stomach upset, diarrhoea, loss of appetite, headache and skin rash. Devil's claw may also interact with anti-clotting drugs such as aspirin, painkillers, heart drugs and antacids. Do not use devil's claw if you have a stomach ulcer or gallstones or if you are pregnant or breastfeeding.

Safety rating: Amber

Evening primrose oil (EPO)

What it is: EPO is derived from the seeds of the evening primrose plant.

Beneficial effects: It improves the pain and morning stiffness of RA.

How it works: The active ingredients are two types of omega-6 essential fatty acids – linolenic acid (LA) and gamma-linolenic acid (GLA). LA is used in the body to make a type of prostaglandin that helps to regulate pain and inflammation and GLA is thought to block inflammation by acting on certain inflammatory cells.

Evidence of effectiveness: In one RCT, 49 people with RA took either 6 g of EPO, 6 g of EPO with fish oil or placebo tablets daily for 12 months. They were asked to take their usual dose of NSAIDs, e.g. ibuprofen, for the first three months, but after that to reduce or stop taking them in response to their symptoms. Two of those taking EPO withdrew because they suffered from nausea and diarrhoea but, after 12 months, 94 per cent of those taking EPO and 93 per cent of those taking EPO with fish oil reported significant improvements in pain and morning stiffness, compared to just 30 per cent of those on the placebo. In another RCT, 40 RA sufferers took 6 g of either EPO or olive oil daily for six months. Four out of the 19 people taking EPO withdrew because of nausea, flu-like symptoms or worsening disease symptoms but, at the end of the trial, those taking EPO reported a significant improvement in morning stiffness compared to those taking olive oil, although there was no difference in terms of pain reduction and disease severity.

Effectiveness score: 3 (for RA)

Safety: There are no major safety concerns, but people with epilepsy are advised against taking EPO, as it can trigger seizures. Common adverse effects include nausea, diarrhoea, bloating and skin rash.

Safety rating: Green

Fish oils

What they are: Fish body oils are obtained from the tissues of oily fish like salmon, mackerel and sardines. Fish liver oils are derived from the livers of cod, halibut or shark.

Beneficial effects: They reduce joint inflammation and lower the risk of heart attacks and stroke in people with inflammatory forms of arthritis. Fish liver oils also help to keep bones and joints healthy.

How they work: The active ingredients are long-chain fatty acids, eicosapentaenoic acid and docosahexaenoic acid, all of which the body uses to make anti-inflammatory prostaglandins (both fish body oil and fish liver oil are good sources of the latter two acids). They are also thought to reduce the production of inflammatory substances by white blood cells and to reduce cholesterol levels in the blood. A study published in *Nature* (a weekly science journal) in 2009 suggested that, as well as producing anti-inflammatory prostaglandins, fish oils might be involved in another mechanism: it claimed that the body converts a component of fish oil into another chemical called resolvin D2 and that this chemical also reduces inflammation. The vitamin A that fish liver oils contain has antioxidant effects and the vitamin D that they provide helps to keep bones strong and also appears to have a role in keeping cartilage healthy.

Evidence of effectiveness: Several RCTs suggest that fish body oil can reduce joint pain and the number of swollen and tender joints in RA, as well as the length of time that morning stiffness and fatigue lasts. In an RCT involving 97 RA sufferers, the group who took capsules containing both cod liver oil and fish body oil had a modest reduction in pain compared to those who took a placebo. They also needed to take fewer NSAIDs. An RCT where participants with OA were given fish liver oil or olive oil did not find any significant difference between the two groups in terms of pain and disability. Recent research by Professor Bruce Caterson at Cardiff University suggests that fish liver oils may prevent OA both by blocking inflammatory responses and by helping to prevent cartilage being destroyed and bones rubbing together.

However, the overall evidence regarding the effectiveness of fish oils for OA has been deemed inconclusive.

Effectiveness score: 1 (fish liver oil for OA)

Effectiveness score: 5 (fish body oil for RA)

Safety: Omega-3 essential fatty acids can interact with blood-thinning drugs, such as warfarin. Fish liver oils (e.g. cod liver oil) also contain vitamin D, which many people in the UK are deficient in, because the major source is sunlight, and vitamin A. A shortage of vitamin D may be linked to the development of arthritis (see Action 12 in Chapter 3), so taking cod liver oil may be beneficial. However, it is advisable not to take fish liver oil if you take a multivitamin or if you eat liver regularly, as any excess of these vitamins is stored in the liver and too much can be harmful. Pregnant women should not take fish liver oils, as vitamin A can cause birth defects. A vegetarian alternative is flaxseed oil, but the body obtains less eicosapentaenoic acid and docosahexaenoic acid from plant sources.

Safety rating: Green

Choosing a fish oil supplement

Note: Experts recommend choosing a supplement containing sufficient amounts of long-chain fatty acids. Many don't provide enough to be of benefit, so look for one containing 500–600 mg of eicosapentaenoic acid or docosahexaenoic acid.

Ginger

What it is: A plant native to China, South East Asia, West Africa and the Caribbean. Herbal supplements are derived from the plant's root.

Beneficial effects: It reduces the pain and disability caused by OA.

How it works: Research suggests that ginger can reduce the activity of various chemicals involved in joint inflammation and pain, including prostaglandins (hormone-like substances involved in inflammation) and leukotrienes (substances involved in immune response). One of the active ingredients is salicylate, which the body converts into salicylic acid, a component of aspirin.

Evidence of effectiveness: Three RCTs have investigated the effectiveness of ginger in the treatment of people with OA. In a study published in *Osteoarthritis and Cartilage* in 2000, 67 participants with OA received either 170 mg of ginger extract, 400 mg ibuprofen tablets, or a placebo three times daily. Those using ginger or ibuprofen had less pain and needed fewer painkillers than those taking the placebo, although the ginger was less effective than the ibuprofen. In another trial published in *Arthritis and Rheumatism* in 2001, 29 people with OA in the knee received either 250 mg of ginger or placebo capsules four times daily for three months. During the following three months, the treatments were then swapped, so that those who had initially received the ginger were given the placebo, and vice versa. At the end of the first three months, the participants taking ginger had significantly less pain and disability than those taking the placebo, but at the end of the second phase, no significant difference was detected. In a third trial, 247 participants with OA in the knee randomly received either 255 mg of ginger capsules or placebo capsules twice daily. After six months of treatment,

63 per cent of the group taking ginger experienced a significant reduction in knee pain, compared to 50 per cent of those taking the placebo.

Effectiveness score: 3 (for OA)

Safety: Ginger is generally safe to use. The adverse effects are usually minor – the most common being an upset stomach and an irritated mouth. To help avoid this, don't take large amounts of raw ginger on an empty stomach. Also, it might increase the risk of bleeding if taken with anticoagulants (drugs that prevent blood clots – such as warfarin and rivaroxaban).

Safety rating: Green

Glucosamine (sulphate and hydrochloride)

What it is: Glucosamine is a type of sugar occurring naturally in the body. The glucosamine sulphate used in supplements is usually derived from the shells of crab, lobster or shrimp, or is produced synthetically from plant sources.

Beneficial effects: It delays cartilage loss and rebuilds cartilage.

How it works: Glucosamine is used by the body to produce and repair joint cartilage and improve the cushioning action of synovial fluid.

Evidence of effectiveness: A review in 2005 of 20 RCTs involving OA sufferers concluded that glucosamine sulphate was more effective than a placebo in improving joint function and relieving pain. However, the further review in 2010 (mentioned above under 'Chondroitin sulphate') concluded that taking glucosamine (alone or with chondroitin) didn't lead to a clinically meaningful reduction in joint pain or change any clinical aspects of the joint.

Effectiveness score: Glucosamine sulphate: 2 (for OA); Glucosamine hydrochloride: 1 (for OA).

Safety: There are few side effects from taking glucosamine sulphate or hydrochloride, although occasionally mild stomach upsets such as nausea or diarrhoea, headache and skin rash have been reported. If you are susceptible to an upset stomach, take glucosamine with food. Animal research pointed to the possibility that glucosamine sulphate or hydrochloride might cause high blood sugar, but two extensive human trials reported that the supplement had no effect on blood sugar levels, in fact it sometimes even lowered them. The current advice is that, if you take this supplement for long periods and have any concerns, you should have your blood sugar level checked. Diabetics should speak to their doctor before taking glucosamine sulphate.

Safety rating: Green

Shellfish allergy alert

Anyone with a shellfish allergy should check the label before taking this supplement – you can buy glucosamine for vegetarians, which does not contain shellfish (see Useful Products). Glucosamine may interact with warfarin, so if you are taking warfarin, inform your doctor or pharmacist before taking it.

Green-lipped mussel

What it is: A supplement derived from a mussel native to New Zealand.

Beneficial effects: It reduces pain and improves joint function.

How it works: It contains omega-3 fatty acids that help to maintain joint health.

Evidence of effectiveness: A recent review of four RCTs concluded that three trials had shown that green-lipped mussel supplements were more beneficial than placebo capsules. Reported benefits included reduced pain, improved functioning and quality of life when taken alongside painkillers such as paracetamol, or NSAIDs. The fourth trial compared the effects of two types of green-lipped mussel supplement – an oil and a powder. Of the participants, 73 per cent of those taking the oil and 87 per cent of those taking the powder showed significant improvements.

Effectiveness score: 3 (for OA)

Safety: Occasionally there may be nausea or flatulence. Do not take green-lipped mussel if you are allergic to shellfish.

Safety rating: Green

Indian frankincense

What it is: A plant extract used in Ayurvedic medicine. Its other names include *Boswellia serrata*, resin, olibanum, African elemi and *Boswellia serrata* gum resins.

Beneficial effects: It reduces pain and improves flexibility and mobility in people with OA of the knee.

How it works: It blocks the production of inflammatory substances.

Evidence of effectiveness: Four RCTs have investigated the use of Indian frankincense in treating osteoarthritis of the knee. In one RCT in 2003, 30 participants with OA of the knee took either 333 mg Indian frankincense capsules or placebo tablets three times a day. After eight weeks, those who took the Indian frankincense reported a moderate improvement in pain, knee flexibility and the distance they were able to walk. In another RCT in 2007, 66 participants with OA of the knee took either 333 mg of Indian frankincense, or the NSAID valdecoxib. Both groups had an improvement in levels of pain, stiffness and mobility. These beneficial effects took longer to appear in those taking Indian frankincense, but they lasted for longer after the treatment stopped. The overall evidence from the four RCTs suggests Indian frankincense may be beneficial to people with knee osteoarthritis.

Effectiveness score: 3 (for OA)

Safety: A daily dose of 1 g is safe, but higher doses can have serious adverse effects on the liver. Minor stomach upsets are occasionally experienced.

Safety rating: Green

Methylsulfonylmethane (MSM)

What it is: MSM is a substance that contains sulphur and is found in fresh raw foods such as fruit, vegetables and meat.

Beneficial effects: It reduces joint pain and swelling and improves general functioning in osteoarthritis sufferers.

How it works: Studies show that MSM has anti-inflammatory and antioxidant effects. Also, the sulphur in MSM is used to produce collagen and glucosamine, which are essential for healthy bones and joints. It's also involved in making antibodies, which are part of the immune system.

Evidence of effectiveness: Three RCTs have looked at MSM's effectiveness as an osteoarthritis treatment.

In one trial, once a day for 12 weeks, 118 participants with knee osteoarthritis randomly received 1.5 g glucosamine, or 1.5 g MSM capsules, or both, or placebos. Participants who took

MSM or glucosamine reported a significant reduction in joint pain and swelling compared to those who took a placebo, with glucosamine having the most effect on joint swelling. Those who took both glucosamine and MSM had the biggest improvement in both pain and swelling and the best joint function.

In another RCT where 50 knee osteoarthritis sufferers took either 6 g MSM capsules or placebo capsules for 12 weeks, only 25 per cent of those on MSM found an improvement in pain and physical function, compared to those who took the placebo. There was no improvement in stiffness.

In the third trial 60 knee osteoarthritis sufferers randomly took either 3.375 g MSM capsules or placebo capsules once daily for 12 weeks. Those taking MSM experienced an improvement in pain and general functional well-being compared to those who took the placebo, but had no improvement in knee function (e.g. when walking or climbing stairs). Arthritis Research UK concluded that there's a small amount of evidence that MSM has a moderate beneficial effect on joint pain and swelling and general functioning in osteoarthritis sufferers, and that the beneficial effect is greater when it is taken with glucosamine.

Effectiveness score: 2 (for OA)

Safety: As a short-term treatment (three months), MSM is well tolerated, even in high doses, but the long-term side effects of MSM aren't known. Only mild side effects have been reported – most commonly gastrointestinal discomfort. No drug interactions have been noted.

Safety rating: Green

Pine bark extracts (Pycnogenol)

What it is: An extract from French pine. Other names include maritime bark and *Pinus pinaster*.

Beneficial effects: It reduces pain, stiffness and swelling and improves mobility in OA.

How it works: It contains bioflavonoids that are anti-inflammatory and antioxidant.

Evidence of effectiveness: In one RCT, 156 people with OA took 100 mg of either pine bark or placebo capsules for three months and were told to take NSAIDs when they needed to. At the end of the trial, those taking the pine bark had a 56 per cent reduction in pain, compared to just ten per cent of those taking the placebo; their use of NSAIDs dropped by 58 per cent, compared to just one per cent among the placebo group and, probably as a result of this, they had fewer gastrointestinal symptoms. In a second trial, 100 people with mild knee osteoarthritis were randomly selected to receive either 150 mg pycnogenol or a placebo for three months. Those who took pycnogenol reported an improvement in function and less pain compared to the group taking the placebo, who found no improvement.

Effectiveness score: 3 (for OA)

Safety: No serious side effects have been reported. Minor side effects include an upset stomach and headache.

Safety rating: Green

Rose hip

What it is: A species of wild rose native to parts of Europe, Asia and Africa. The medicinal compound is taken from the fruits that appear after the flowers have died.

Beneficial effects: It relieves pain and stiffness in both OA and RA.

How it works: The active ingredients are thought to include the antioxidants anthocyanins (plant pigments that give rose hips their red colour) and polyphenols, as well as a sugary fatty acid known as GOPO, and vitamin C. These ingredients are thought to prevent joint damage and relieve inflammation.

Evidence of effectiveness: A review of three studies by researchers from Frederiksberg Hospital in Denmark, the University of California and the University of Copenhagen provided sound evidence that rose hip powder can relieve the pain of OA. A total of 306 participants took 5 g of either a powder made from *Rosa canina* (a wild rose hip) or a placebo for an average period of three months. The combined results of these studies suggested that taking *Rosa canina* cut pain levels to about a third of those experienced in the placebo group. People using the powder were also less likely to use other painkillers and reported less stiffness. Another study published in 2008 by the Department of Human Nutrition and Health in Basel, Switzerland, reported that rose hip extracts may regenerate joints affected by arthritis. The study measured the effects of different doses of GOPO, extracted from rose hips, on human cartilage cells. Researchers concluded that GOPO blocked the production of immune cells involved in the destruction of joints and promoted the production of collagen. Other research in Germany in 2007 involving 74, mainly female, RA sufferers showed that those taking a rose hip supplement alongside their usual medication had 40 per cent less joint pain than those taking a placebo with medication. The group taking the rose hip supplement also had improved mobility.

Effectiveness score: 3 for OA and 2 for RA

Safety: Any side effects are usually mild, but can include allergic reactions, diarrhoea, constipation and heartburn.

Safety rating: Green

SAMe (S-Adenosyl methionine)

What it is: SAMe is a chemical compound found naturally in the body that is derived from methionine, an amino acid found in high-protein foods, and adenosine triphosphate (ATP), a substance involved in the production of energy in the body.

Beneficial effects: It reduces pain and improves joint function in OA and it reduces tenderness and depression in fibromyalgia.

How it works: It stimulates the production of two major components of cartilage – collagen and proteoglycans. It also has painkilling properties.

Evidence of effectiveness: A review of the combined data from 11 RCTs investigating the effectiveness of SAMe in the treatment of OA concluded that it had a similar effect to NSAIDs in terms of improving joint function and reducing pain. Data from ten of the trials comparing SAMe to aspirin or an NSAID suggested that those taking SAMe were 58 per cent less likely to suffer from adverse effects. The daily dose used in these studies ranged from 400 mg to 1,600 mg. Another trial in 2004 compared the effectiveness of SAMe to celecoxib (a type of medication known as a COX-2 inhibitor). It reported that, although SAMe took longer to have an effect, it was as good as celecoxib at relieving pain and improving physical functioning after 16 weeks of use. Three out of four RCTs investigating the role of SAMe in the treatment of fibromyalgia reported that SAMe was more effective than a placebo in reducing the number of tender points and/or the degree of tenderness felt as well as the symptoms of depression. The fourth RCT concluded that SAMe was no better than a placebo in reducing fibromyalgia symptoms.

Effectiveness score: 4 for OA and 2 for fibromyalgia

Safety: Occasional mild side effects include nausea, headache, dry mouth, upset stomach and restlessness. More severe side effects – usually in people with depression – include anxiety and mania. SAMe can increase the risk of bleeding if taken with blood-thinning medications like aspirin, heparin and warfarin, so if you are taking any such medications, talk to your GP or pharmacist before taking it.

Safety rating: Green

Sigesbeckia

What it is: Sigesbeckia, nicknamed 'pig pungent weed' because of its unpleasant smell, is a small shrub native to eastern Asia. Extracts from the leaves, flowers and stems have been used for hundreds of years in Chinese medicine for the relief of muscle and joint pain.

Beneficial effects: Sigesbeckia eases muscle and joint aches and pains.

How it works: It has an anti-inflammatory effect.

Evidence of effectiveness: Based on traditional use only.

Effectiveness score: Not yet rated by Arthritis Research UK; however in 2015 it became the first traditional Chinese herbal medicine to be approved by the MHRA as an over-the-counter treatment.

Safety: Possible but uncommon side effects include diarrhoea, nausea, vomiting, headaches and dizziness, rash and itching, if you are sensitive to any of the ingredients. Sigesbeckia is not recommended for under 18-year-olds. You should not use this product if you are pregnant or breastfeeding.

Safety rating: Not yet rated by Arthritis Research UK, but according to the MHRA there are no undesirable effects.

Stinging nettle

What it is: A common wild plant that has traditionally been used to treat arthritis and rheumatic disorders.

Beneficial effects: It reduces pain and disability in OA.

How it works: The leaves are rich in vitamins and minerals, natural anti-inflammatories and natural painkillers. When a nettle stings the skin, it injects various chemicals, including histamine and serotonin, which are thought to stimulate pain in the nerve cells and have a counterirritant effect that overrides arthritis pain.

Evidence of effectiveness: Two RCTs – one in 2000 and the other in 2008 – evaluated the effectiveness of stinging nettle as a treatment for people with OA. The first trial lasted for three months and involved 27 people with OA pain at the base of the thumb. Participants were randomly asked to apply either a stinging nettle leaf or a placebo leaf to the affected area daily for a week. After five weeks they were asked to apply the other type of leaf for one week. The people using the stinging nettle leaves experienced significantly less pain and disability in the first week after treatment than those using the placebo leaves. After that, the benefits gradually disappeared. The second trial lasted for one week and involved 42 people with OA in the knee who were randomly asked to apply either stinging nettle leaves or leaves from another nettle to their knees. After one week, both groups reported a mild but insignificant reduction in pain. On the basis of these results, Arthritis Research UK gave stinging nettle a low effectiveness score. However, it could be argued that the first trial did show promising results and in both cases nettle leaves were only applied for one week. Perhaps longer trials need to be done to determine whether this common weed can benefit arthritis sufferers.

Effectiveness score: 1 (for OA)
Safety: Causes minor short-term irritation when applied to the skin.
Safety rating: Green

Make your own nettle tea

If you'd like to try using stinging nettle, but don't like the idea of being stung, you can buy a stinging nettle tincture or nettle tea, or make your own nettle tea with the following simple recipe. To avoid being stung, wear gloves when collecting the nettles and preparing the tea. Rinse 50 g of young, fresh nettle leaves in lukewarm water and then soak in 500 ml of boiling water for about ten minutes. Strain and drink either hot or cold. Sweeten with honey if desired. Bear in mind, however, that there is only anecdotal evidence that taking a nettle tincture or tea relieves arthritis symptoms.

Handy tip: Use a coffee cafetière to make herbal tea quickly and easily. Place the herbs in the cafetière before adding the boiling water. Replace the lid and leave to brew, then press down the plunger and pour.

Supplement selector

Use the table below to help you select a suitable supplement for your symptoms.

Condition	Supplement/s with consistent evidence of effectiveness	Supplement/s with some evidence of effectiveness	Supplement/s with little evidence of effectiveness
Osteoarthritis	Capsaicin gel, Indian frankincense, SAMe (S-Adenosyl methionine), Sigesbeckia	Chondroitin sulphate, devil's claw, ginger, glucosamine sulphate, green-lipped mussel, pine bark extracts, rose hip, stinging nettle, fish liver oil, glucosamine hydrochloride	
Rheumatoid arthritis	Fish body oil	Borage seed oil, evening primrose oil, rose hip	
Fibromyalgia			Capsaicin gel, SAMe (S-Adenosyl methionine)

Chapter 5

Arthritis and Emotions

Like many other health conditions, it seems that arthritis can be triggered or made worse by stress. Living with arthritis can be stressful, which leads to a vicious cycle of emotional symptoms, such as anxiety and depression, and physical pain. In a survey of 232 people with RA, around 39 per cent said that their symptoms left them severely anxious and/or depressed, whilst a further 41 per cent said that they were moderately anxious and/or depressed. This chapter looks at what stress is and how it may be involved in OA, RA and other inflammatory forms of arthritis. Stress management and relaxation techniques are suggested to help prevent and relieve flare-ups and reduce tension and anxiety.

What is stress?

Stress is basically the way the mind and body respond to situations and pressures that leave us feeling inadequate or unable to cope. One person may cope well in a situation that another might find stressful; it's all down to the individual's perception of it and their ability to deal with it.

How does stress affect the body?

The brain reacts to stress by preparing the body to either stay put and face the perceived threat, or to escape from it. It does this by releasing hormones – chemical messengers –including adrenaline, noradrenaline and cortisol into the bloodstream. These speed up the heart rate and breathing patterns and can induce sweating. Glucose and fatty acid levels in the blood rise, to provide a burst of energy to deal with the threat. This is called the 'fight or flight' response.

Nowadays, the situations that induce the stress response are unlikely to necessitate either of these reactions. Those that continue for a long period of time, for example long-term unemployment, illness or an unhappy relationship, mean that stress hormone levels remain high, thereby increasing the risk of major health conditions such as coronary heart disease and stroke, as well as autoimmune disorders, such as RA. Other psychological and physical symptoms include irritability, poor concentration, anxiety, depression, headaches, skin problems, allergies, poor appetite or overeating, indigestion, IBS (irritable bowel syndrome) and palpitations, so it's important to find ways to reduce and deal with stress.

How is stress involved in arthritis symptoms?

Research suggests that long-term exposure to stress hormones can affect the immune system and provoke inflammation in the body, which can trigger or exacerbate RA and other inflammatory forms of arthritis.

Also, when we are stressed we tend to tense our muscles – especially those in the neck, shoulders and arms, which can put a strain on the joints and both cause and worsen pain from all types of arthritis.

18 Identify your stress triggers

There are basically three things you can do to manage stress: avoid it, reduce it and relieve it. But first, you need to identify what makes you feel stressed.

Keep a stress diary

Over a couple of weeks, note down the details of situations, times, places and people that make you feel stressed. Once you've identified these, think about each one and ask yourself: 'Can I avoid it?' For example, if you find driving to work during the rush hour stressful, perhaps you can avoid it by starting or finishing work a little earlier or later. If you cannot avoid it, you can usually reduce the level of stress you experience by changing your attitude towards a situation or by taking practical steps to help you cope better. You can also relieve the effects of stress by practising relaxation techniques and doing things that help you unwind.

Don't sweat the small stuff!

As well as recognising the external factors that make you feel stressed, consider whether some aspects of your personality are also to blame. Are you a perfectionist who is never satisfied with your achievements and lifestyle? Constantly feeling that who you are and what you have aren't good enough can lead to unrealistic expectations, discontent and unnecessary pressure. In his best-selling book *Don't Sweat the Small Stuff*, Dr Richard Carlson urges us to remind ourselves that 'life is OK the way it is, right now'. Adopting this attitude immediately reduces stress and induces calm.

You'll never reach the end of your 'to-do list'

Workaholism is another factor that tends to be linked with perfectionism – a 'perfect' home and lifestyle have to be paid for. Whilst working hard for what you want in life is commendable, some people work such long hours that they don't have time to enjoy what they have. If you're constantly driven to get everything done, and think you'll feel calm and relaxed once everything on your 'to-do list' is completed, think again! What tends to happen is that as you complete tasks, you add new ones to your list, so you never get to the end of it. It's a fact of life that there will always be tasks to be completed. Overdoing things can also make your arthritis symptoms worse, so it's especially important that you pace yourself.

Don't worry!

Worrying about events that haven't even happened can bring on the stress response, as your body can't differentiate between what has actually happened and what you imagine happening. For example, if you fear that your arthritis might get worse or if you worry about paying your mortgage, your body will produce stress hormones, even if your condition doesn't actually deteriorate or you don't lose your home. Although it's hard not to worry about the things that might go wrong in your life, it's better for your health if you can make a conscious decision not to worry about things that haven't happened yet.

19 Change your attitude

When difficult situations do come along, changing your attitude towards them can reduce the amount of stress they cause, because it is your interpretation of the event, not the event itself, that elicits your emotional response. When something bad happens, instead of thinking about how awful the situation is, try to find something positive about it if you can. Try to find positive solutions to your problems, or view them as opportunities for personal growth. For example, being made redundant initially seems like a negative event but, if you view it as an opportunity to retrain and start a new career doing something you really enjoy, it can become a catalyst for positive change. Researchers at the University of Bath found that people with chronic arthritis who had a positive attitude towards life sufferered less pain and disability than those whose outlook was negative.

20 Live in the moment

Living in the moment, or practising mindfulness, has been shown to reduce stress levels. It involves giving all of your attention to the here and now, rather than worrying about the past or future, and has its roots in Buddhism. It's based on the philosophy that you can't alter the past, or foretell the future, but you can influence what's happening in your life right now. By living fully in the present, you can perform to the best of your ability, whereas worrying about the past and future can hamper how you function now and can increase your stress levels unnecessarily.

Living in this way means your experience of life is richer, because instead of doing things on autopilot, all of your senses will be fully engaged in what you are doing. Imagine going for a walk in the park whilst being so preoccupied with worries about the future, or regrets about the past, that you don't even notice your surroundings. Then think how much more pleasurable and relaxing the experience would be if you took the time to absorb the sights, sounds and smells around you. When you focus on the here and now, you will find yourself appreciating the simple things in your life more.

Mindfulness is also about being happy with your life as it is now, rather than wishing things were different. Octavius Black, co-author of *The Mind Gym: Give Me Time*, suggests that we should 'make today be tomorrow's happy memories'. Adopting this attitude towards life will immediately lower your stress levels. If you find it hard to focus on the present, try keeping a daily diary.

21 Simplify your life

If you feel that your life is spiralling out of control with too many demands from work, your home, your partner, your family and friends, maybe it's time to simplify your life. If you regularly feel under pressure and stressed because of a lack of time, try reviewing how you use it. Keep a diary for a few days to see how you spend your time and then decide which activities you can cut out or reduce to make more time for the things that are most important to you. Try saying no to the non-essential tasks you don't have time for, or just don't want to do. It's a little word, but it can dramatically reduce your stress levels. If you find it hard to say no, then perhaps you need to develop your assertiveness skills.

Cut down on having and concentrate on being

The psychologist and author Oliver James warns that our preoccupation with acquiring more and more material goods means that we end up working longer hours and becoming tired and stressed. He advises that, before buying something, you should ask yourself whether you need it, or simply want it, and that when you do this you will soon realise that you are spending more than you need to. He advocates cutting down on having and concentrating on being.

Slow down

Many of us are living our lives at a faster and faster pace, perhaps juggling a full-time job with a relationship, family commitments and a social life. As a result, we feel a constant sense of urgency in our daily lives as we race from one task to another. This constant feeling of pressure fuels our impatience when we have to wait in a queue or a traffic jam or the bus or train is late. Octavius Black says we need to accept that we will never have enough time to do everything. He believes that, in order to enjoy the moment, we need to slow down, perhaps viewing situations such as queuing or travel delays as welcome thinking or reading time, rather than allowing impatience and frustration to raise our stress levels unnecessarily.

Prioritise

When you have a long 'to-do list', number tasks in terms of urgency and importance and carry them out in that order.

Delegate

Perfectionism can also lead to a need to control – you convince yourself that no one else can meet your high standards, so you do everything yourself. This inevitably leads to physical and mental overload. The solution is to accept that you can't know and do everything, so you need to learn to listen to other people's ideas and opinions and to delegate. Ask your partner and children to help with domestic tasks and accept any offers of help at work. This is especially important if you are finding it hard to cope during an arthritis flare-up.

Clear away clutter

If a bulging wardrobe, heaving shelves and overflowing cupboards are getting you down, make your life simpler and less stressful by getting rid of unnecessary clutter around your home. You'll save time and energy, because you'll find things more quickly in a clutter-free environment and your mental clarity will improve, because ridding yourself of physical clutter clears mental clutter. If you haven't worn, read or used an item for two years or more, give it to a charity shop, sell it on ebay or bin it. If you can't bear to get rid of it, store it in the loft, then make it a rule that if you haven't thought about using the item within six months, it is time to part with it. If you have a lot of possessions to sort out, ask your partner, a family member or a friend to help you. You'll be amazed at how much happier and less stressed you will feel after a good clear-out.

22 Assert yourself

If you feel you often hide your true feelings instead of expressing them, and give in to others so that you don't hurt or upset them or to gain their approval, you might benefit from brushing up your assertiveness skills. Some studies suggest a direct link between hiding feelings and the onset of arthritis: Dr Ronald Lamont-Havers, former Medical Director of the Arthritis and Rheumatism Foundation, and researchers at the University of Southern California, have suggested that stress from bottling up emotions such as anger and fear often accompanies the beginning of arthritis.

Do you regularly allow others to manipulate you into doing things you don't want to do? Being assertive empowers you to say what you want, feel and need, calmly and confidently, without being aggressive or hurting others. The following techniques will help you to express your emotions and remain in control of your life, by doing things because you want to, rather than to please other people.

- Demonstrate ownership of your thoughts, feelings and behaviour by using 'I' rather than 'we', 'you' or 'it'. For example, rather than saying 'You make me angry', try something like 'I feel angry when you...' This is less antagonising to the other person.

- When you have a choice whether to do something or not, say 'won't' rather than 'can't' to show that you've made an active decision, rather than suggesting that something or someone has stopped you. Say 'choose to' instead of 'have to' and 'could' rather than 'should', to indicate that you have a choice. For example: 'I won't be going out tonight' rather than 'I can't go out tonight,' or 'I could go out tonight, but I've chosen to stay in.'

- When you feel that your needs aren't being considered, state what you want calmly and clearly, repeating it until the other person shows they've heard and understood what you've said.

- When making a request, identify exactly what it is you want and what you're prepared to settle for. Choose positive, assertive words, as outlined above. For example: 'I would like you to help me tidy the kitchen and I'd really appreciate it if you could empty the kitchen bin.'

- When refusing a request, speak calmly but firmly, giving the reason or reasons for your refusal without apologising. Repeat if you need to. For example: 'I won't be able to babysit for you tonight because I'm feeling really tired after being at work all day.'

- When you disagree with someone, say so using the word 'I'. Explain why you disagree, but acknowledge the other person's right to have a different viewpoint. For example: 'I don't agree that the service in that restaurant is poor – our meal was only late last time we visited because it was very busy, but I can understand why you think that.'

㉓ Seek support

Arthritis can be an isolating condition that leaves many sufferers feeling that no one understands what they are experiencing. Making contact with fellow sufferers who are dealing with the same symptoms as you may help you to overcome these feelings. The organisations listed here offer the opportunity to do just that; further information and contact details can be found in the Directory at the end of the book.

Arthritis Care is a UK charity that aims to empower arthritis sufferers by providing high-quality information and support. The charity offers a free, confidential helpline and an online discussion forum where arthritis sufferers can both find and offer support. You can also sign up to free e-updates, which contain the latest news about arthritis and links to further information and features. There is also a network of over 300 Arthritis Care groups across the UK. These groups offer regular events, meetings and support for people with arthritis. You can find your nearest group on the regional pages of the website.

Arthritis Forum is a group and website offering help, support and friendship to fellow sufferers. The forum states that it aims 'to concentrate on the day-to-day business of having arthritis, how it affects our lives and how we deal with the challenges it throws up'. Membership of the online forum, where you can take part in discussions about living with arthritis, is free and there is also a Personal Stories section where you can tell other people about your experiences of living with arthritis.

Health Boards is a website that offers online community message boards on a variety of health conditions, including arthritis.

The National Rheumatoid Arthritis Society (NRAS) offers a helpline and a members' forum, as well as a network of volunteers who themselves have RA and who provide peer support to fellow sufferers. There are also several NRAS groups around the UK that meet regularly to offer a range of informative and social activities that increase knowledge of the condition and reduce the isolation that some sufferers feel.

NHS Talk provides blogs and forums on medical conditions, including various types of arthritis. The blogs provide personal insights from patients, carers and medical professionals about managing a particular medical condition and the forums enable people to request advice and share experiences and information.

Patient UK Experience is a forum provided by Patient UK, a website offering health information 'as provided by GPs and nurses to patients during consultations', where you can read about others' experiences of medical conditions – including various types of arthritis – medications, treatments and services, and share your own.

Help is at hand

If you feel you can't deal with life's stresses on your own, don't be afraid to seek professional help. Your first port of call should be your doctor, as he or she should be able to offer advice, and possibly refer you to a counsellor.

The Stress Management Society offers further guidance on dealing with stress, including 'desk yoga' and 'desk massage' techniques you can practise at work, and a creative visualisation you can do whenever you have a few minutes to yourself. See the Directory at the end of the book for contact details.

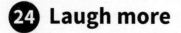 Laugh more

Laughter is a great stress reliever. A good belly laugh seems to reduce the stress hormones cortisol and adrenaline and trigger mood-boosting serotonin levels. People who see the funny side of life appear to have a reduced risk of the health problems associated with stress. It is also thought that chemicals released when we laugh, such as endorphins and enkephalins, can help to ease the pain of arthritis. Research at the University of Bath and Royal National Hospital for Rheumatic Diseases, Bath, found that patients with chronic arthritis who were able to laugh experienced less pain. So make time to watch your favourite comedies and comedians and be around people who make you laugh. Or visit websites like www.laughlab.co.uk or www.ahajokes.com whenever you feel like a good giggle!

25 Do something purely for pleasure

Spend time each day doing something purely for pleasure, whether it's enjoying a long soak in a warm, scented bath, sitting down with a glass of wine and a good book, listening to your favourite music, or going to the cinema. Doing something you really enjoy will help to take your mind off your arthritis symptoms and any domestic and work pressures.

26 Get physical!

Regular exercise is a great antidote to stress, because it enables the body to use the stress hormones whose purpose is to provide the extra energy needed to run away from our aggressors, or to stay put and fight. It also triggers the release of endorphins, which act as natural painkillers and antidepressants. For more information about the best types of exercise for arthritis sufferers, see Chapter 6.

27 Enjoy ecotherapy

Researchers at Essex University say that ecotherapy (engaging with nature) offers both mental and physical health benefits. Whether through an active pursuit such as walking or gardening or a passive one such as admiring the view, being close to nature has been shown to reduce stress and ease muscular tension. Experts claim that the higher levels of negative ions near areas with running water, trees and mountains may play a part. Others suggest that the success of ecotherapy is down to 'biophilia' – the theory that we all have an innate affinity with nature and that our 'disconnection' from it is the cause of stress and mental health problems. Studies in the Netherlands and Japan suggest that people living in or near 'green' areas enjoy a longer and healthier life than those living in urban environments.

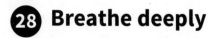 28 Breathe deeply

When we're stressed, our breathing tends to become shallow, or we hold our breath without realising it. Slow, deep breathing has been shown to reduce the heart rate, relax muscles and release tension. Focusing on your breathing helps to take your mind off any discomfort you are feeling. So the next time you're stressed or in pain, try taking control of your breathing.

Try this simple breathing exercise:

- Inhale slowly through your nostrils to a count of five, allowing your stomach to expand.

- Hold for a count of five.

- Breathe out slowly through your nose to a count of five, whilst slowly flattening your stomach.

- Repeat up to ten times.

29 Practise muscle relaxation

When your joints are painful, the natural response is to tense your muscles, which leads to more pain. Progressive muscle relaxation helps to release tension from the muscles, thus alleviating discomfort. And, according to Richard Hilliard, director of the

Relaxation for Living Institute (RFL), it's impossible to have an anxious mind when your muscles are relaxed. The Institute's website offers advice on relaxation and stress management, as well as a guided deep relaxation as an MP3 download that you can purchase. See the Directory for details.

Try following these steps whenever you feel tense and anxious.

- Take a deep breath and then create tension in your face by clenching your teeth and screwing up your eyes tightly, then relax and breathe out.

- Take a deep breath, then lift the muscles in your shoulders, tense them for a few seconds and then relax, dropping your shoulders and releasing the tension as you breathe out.

- Take a deep breath, then clench your fists and tense the muscles in your arms, hold for a few seconds then release and breathe out.

- Next, breathe in, while tensing the muscles in your buttocks and your legs, including the thighs and calves, hold, and then release as you breathe out.

- Finally, take a deep breath and clench your toes and tense your feet, hold, and then release and breathe out.

30 Meditate

Research suggests that meditation lowers stress. There are various meditation techniques, but here is a simple one that can be practised whenever you have a few moments to yourself – even whilst on the bus or train!

Close your eyes and focus on your breathing. As you inhale slowly and deeply through your nose, expand your stomach, hold for a few seconds, before drawing in your stomach, whilst exhaling slowly. Whenever your attention is distracted by a passing thought, return to simply observing your breathing. If you prefer, you can listen to a step-by-step mindfulness meditation at www.stressmanagement.co.uk.

❸❶ Sleep soundly

It is thought that around 80 per cent of OA sufferers, 50 per cent of RA sufferers, 75 per cent of fibromyalgia sufferers and 80 per cent of lupus sufferers have problems sleeping. Lack of sleep increases stress levels and can leave you feeling unable to cope.

The pain of arthritis can make it difficult to sleep soundly, and studies suggest that a lack of sleep increases the release of a type of cytokine (a protein with various roles in the body) that promotes inflammation and therefore aggravates symptoms. Whilst pain can be eased through exercise and the use of NSAIDs, there are other steps you can take to improve your sleep patterns.

To sleep more soundly, try the following:

- Take steps to ease any pain before bedtime. This might include applying a pain-relieving gel or taking appropriate painkillers, taking some gentle exercise, or perhaps asking your partner to gently massage the areas that are painful.

- Get outdoors during the day. Exposure to daylight stops the production of melatonin, the brain chemical that promotes sleep, making it easier for your body to release it at night so that you fall asleep more easily and sleep more soundly.

- Choose foods rich in tryptophan, an amino acid that your body uses to produce serotonin (a brain chemical that's converted into melatonin). Tryptophan-rich foods include bananas, dates, dairy foods, chicken, turkey, rice, oats, wholegrain breads and cereals. Make sure you're neither too hungry nor too full when you go to bed, as both can cause wakefulness.

- Don't drink coffee or cola after 2 p.m., because the stimulant effects of the caffeine they contain can last for hours. Whilst tea contains about half as much caffeine – around 50 mg per cup – it's best not to drink it near bedtime if you have difficulty sleeping. Redbush or herb teas, which are caffeine free, make good alternatives.

- Exercise can help you sleep more soundly, because it encourages your body temperature and metabolism to increase and then fall a few hours later, which promotes sleep. Try not to exercise later than early evening, as exercising too late at night can keep you awake because the body temperature may still be raised at bedtime. Not taking enough exercise can cause sleep problems and restlessness. Even gentle stretching can help you to fall asleep more easily.

- Wind down before bedtime. Develop a regular routine in the evening that allows you to 'put the day to bed'. This could involve watching TV, if you find that relaxing – although it's probably best to avoid watching anything that could prey on your mind later on when you are trying to go to sleep. Other relaxing activities you could do include reading or listening to music.

- Soak in a warm bath at bedtime. Your temperature increases slightly with the warmth and then falls – helping you to drop off. In addition, the warmth can help to relax tense muscles and relieve pain – epecially if you add pain-relieving essential oils, such as rosemary, lavender or chamomile.

- Avoid drinking alcohol at bedtime: although it may relax you at first and help you fall asleep more quickly, it has a stimulant effect, causing you to awaken more often during the night. It's also a diuretic, making nocturnal trips to the toilet more likely. But, if abstinence doesn't help you sleep better, it may be worth indulging in a glass of Cabernet Sauvignon, Merlot or Chianti at bedtime – there's some evidence that these wines improve your sleep patterns, because the grape skins of these varieties are rich in plant melatonin.

- Ensure that your bedroom is cool and dark. Your brain tries to reduce your body temperature at night to slow down your metabolism so, to encourage sleep, aim for a temperature of around 16°C. Darkness stimulates the pineal gland in the brain to produce melatonin.

- Make sure you choose the correct mattress. An easy way to check whether a mattress gives you the right support is to lie on your back and slip a hand under your lower back. There should be just enough space for your hand to fit in the gap between your back and the mattress. If there's no space, the mattress is probably too soft. A bed board beneath the mattress could help. If there's a lot of space, it's likely that it is too hard for you.

- Choose a pillow that will provide support for the neck and head and keep your spine in line with your neck. The Sleep Council advocates using a soft pillow, and Sammy Margo, physiotherapist and author of *The Good Sleep Guide*, suggests it should be fairly flat; though the best pillow height for you depends on the width of your shoulders – if you have narrow shoulders, choose a flatter pillow; if you have broad shoulders, you may need two pillows.

- To help your brain to associate the bedroom with sleep and sex only, avoid having a TV or computer in your bedroom. Watching TV or using a computer last thing at night can overstimulate your brain, making it harder for you to switch off and fall asleep. Also, both TV and computer screens emit bright light that may interfere with the production of melatonin.

- Only go to bed when you feel really sleepy. If you can't drop off within what seems like around 20 minutes, get up and do something you find relaxing, such as reading or listening to calming music. Only return to your bed when you feel drowsy again – this helps to reinforce your brain's connection between your bed and sleep.

- If mulling over problems or a busy schedule the next day stops you from falling asleep, try writing down your concerns or a plan for the day ahead before you go to bed.

Chapter 6

Benefit from Exercise

When you suffer from pain and stiffness on a daily basis, exercise might be the last thing you feel like doing. However, exercise should be an important part of everyone's daily life, especially if you have arthritis, because being inactive increases your risk of being overweight and developing heart disease, certain cancers and osteoporosis. Being overweight puts more strain on your joints and can both cause and worsen arthritis symptoms. RA itself can affect the heart and raise the risk of osteoporosis, and some of the medications commonly prescribed for arthritis, for example steroids, can weaken the bones. Taking regular exercise can help to reduce these risks and improve muscle strength, joint mobility and posture, as well as encourage weight loss, reduce stress levels and even ease pain and stiffness. In a survey of people with OA by Arthritis Care, 57 per cent said that they exercise to help manage their condition.

This chapter offers an overview of the various types of exercise that are especially suitable for people with arthritis and gives advice on how to exercise safely.

What are the benefits of different types of exercise?

Different types of exercise offer specific benefits. For example, low-impact aerobic activities such as walking, swimming and cycling can improve general fitness and strength without putting too much strain on the joints. Gentle stretching exercises like yoga, t'ai chi and Pilates help to loosen up the affected joints, improving flexibility and mobility, and also lengthen the muscles and tendons and increase muscle tone.

What does 'aerobic' mean?

The term 'aerobic' is used to describe exercise that increases the heart rate. It boosts the metabolism, helping to burn calories and control weight, and keeps the heart and bones strong. During aerobic exercise you should feel slightly out of breath and have a faster pulse.

Important exercise dos and don'ts:

- If you have RA, aim to exercise when you feel least tired. Gentle exercise first thing may help to relieve morning stiffness. Exercising early in the evening can help to reduce pain the next morning.

- If you have OA, avoid strenuous exercise, as this may cause further joint damage and pain.

- If you have had joint replacement surgery, avoid high-impact exercise such as running, and don't play contact sports.

- Don't overdo things – aim to gradually build up the amount of time that you exercise. If you are in pain a couple of hours after exercising, you have probably done too much.

- If you experience severe pain in your joints whilst exercising, stop and seek advice from a physiotherapist or your GP.

- If you have RA and one or more joints become painful, warm and swollen whilst exercising, you should stop.

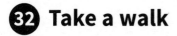 Take a walk

Walking is a great way to exercise if you have arthritis – you can fit it into everyday life and it's free! You can also tailor how far and how quickly you walk to suit your level of mobility and fitness. If you're normally inactive, it's best to build up gradually, perhaps initially walking for ten minutes each day, increasing to 15 minutes and then 20 to 30 minutes. Easy ways to fit more walking into your daily routine include walking to the shops instead of driving or using public transport. Alternatively, you could get off the bus one stop earlier, or park the car further away from your destination. Walking your dog, or a neighbour's, is another way of ensuring you walk more.

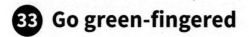 Go green-fingered

Gardening is a weight-bearing exercise and has been deemed more effective than jogging for strengthening bones. Performing light gardening tasks can improve your strength and agility without putting too much strain on your joints, providing you don't overdo things – limit your activity to no more than 30 minutes. Avoid doing one particular task for too long – take a break or do another job so that you use different muscles. Use a lightweight garden hose and garden kneelers to reduce the strain on your muscles and joints. If you must use a watering can, don't overfill it and take care how you lift it, to avoid straining. For more in-depth information on gardening with arthritis see Arthritis Research UK's booklet *Gardening and Arthritis*, which is available on their website (see Directory).

Fit in fitness

If you think you don't have the time to exercise, try being more active in your everyday life; vacuuming the house is a good aerobic exercise that works both the arm and leg muscles. Doing the ironing works the arm muscles and pegging clothes on the washing line gives the whole body a good stretch. Even washing up can help to loosen the finger joints and emptying the dishwasher can stretch arm and core muscles.

---

34 Get in the swim

Swimming is an excellent form of exercise for arthritis sufferers, because the water supports the body's weight, which means it doesn't put much strain on the joints. It both strengthens and stretches the muscles and improves cardiovascular fitness. Also, warm water relaxes the joints and muscles, enabling the joints to move more freely. Swimming may be especially beneficial if you have OA of the hip or knee.

Breaststroke may be unsuitable if you have arthritis in the neck, knees or hips, as it can put too much strain on them. To improve your swimming technique, visit www.swimfit.com, a website that offers animated swimming stroke guides. For information about swimming lessons, visit www.swimtime.org.

35 Try t'ai chi

T'ai chi, described as a 'moving meditation', is an ancient Chinese art that promotes both mental and physical well-being. The movements are slow and controlled, helping to improve strength, flexibility, posture and balance. T'ai chi is popular among arthritis sufferers because it improves fitness and energy levels gently and without strain.

The evidence regarding the effectiveness of t'ai chi in improving arthritis symptoms is mixed. A systematic review of two RCTs and three non-RCTs (i.e. trials where participants are selected to receive a particular treatment) using t'ai chi for people with RA, published in 2007 in the *Journal of Rheumatology*, concluded they had all reported an improvement in quality of life and mood and a reduction in disability. However, the two trials that assessed the effects of t'ai chi on pain did not demonstrate any improvement. The reviewers added that evidence to support the effectiveness of t'ai chi as a treatment for RA was unconvincing overall, because of the poor quality of the trials.

A South Korean study published in the *Journal of Rheumatology* in 2003 involved 43 middle-aged women with OA. Researchers found that women in the group that followed a 12-week t'ai chi programme had less pain and stiffness and improved physical functioning, whereas those in the control group experienced no changes. A trial in 2009 at Tufts University in Massachusetts concluded that t'ai chi was better than general stretching exercises for easing pain and improving mobility in people with OA of the knee. It is possible to learn t'ai chi at home using an instructional DVD (see Directory) but it is probably better to learn how to perform the movements correctly by joining a class – for details of classes near you visit www.taichifinder. co.uk. Many arthritis care groups also run t'ai chi classes.

36 Practise Pilates

Pilates is a low-impact exercise programme devised by the gymnast Joseph H. Pilates to firm the abdominal (core) muscles and generally lengthen and strengthen all of the muscles in the body. In her book *Pilates for Every Body*, the American fitness programme presenter Denise Austin recommends Pilates for OA, saying that it soothes soreness. She claims that the stretches help to keep the joints healthy by pumping vital nutrients to the muscles and tendons and encouraging the production of synovial fluid. She also says that practising Pilates can reduce pain, fatigue and stiffness and improve flexibility. Pilates encourages good posture, which also helps to prevent joint strain, as well as deep, controlled breathing which can help to alleviate tension. Pilates can be practised at home – there are various instructional DVDs available, but it is probably best to join a class initially, to ensure that you adopt the correct posture and perform the exercises properly. Most leisure centres and health clubs now offer Pilates classes. The Body Control Pilates Association provides details of qualified instructors (see Directory).

37 Say 'yes' to yoga

The word yoga comes from the Sanskrit word yuj, which means union. Yogic postures (asanas) and breathing exercises are designed to unite the body, mind and soul. It's a gentle form of exercise that not only strengthens the joints and muscles and increases flexibility and mobility, but also eases aches and pains, improves balance, relieves stress and induces calm, making it ideal for most arthritis sufferers.

There is a growing body of evidence that yoga is beneficial for people with arthritis. A small RCT published in the *Journal of Rheumatology* in 1994 suggested that yoga can improve movement and reduce pain and tenderness in people with OA of the fingers. In another study, published in the *Indian Journal of Physiology and Pharmacology* in 2001, 20 RA sufferers showed improved hand grip strength after practising yoga for 15 days, compared with a control group. Female participants showed a bigger improvement than male participants. A more recent trial involving 30 people with RA, who were divided into two groups, reported that the group that followed an eight-week yoga programme had less joint tenderness and swelling than the sedentary control group. Other studies have suggested that yoga may benefit those with OA in their knees.

Here are some simple yoga exercises that may help to improve arthritis symptoms:

Hand clenches
This yoga exercise is especially good for those with OA or RA in the hands, as it helps to strengthen grip.

1. Adopt a comfortable, seated position, or sit up straight on a chair.

2. Inhale as you lift both arms in front of you to shoulder level, keeping them straight and parallel with the floor.

3. With palms facing down exhale and clench your fists, tucking your thumbs into your fingers.

4. Hold for a few seconds, then open your hands, stretching out your fingers as you inhale.

5. Exhale whilst lowering your arms down to your sides.

6. Repeat the sequence up to eight times.

Wrist circles

Wrist circles loosen up the wrist joints, helping to improve movement.

1. Follow steps 1 to 3 of the fist clench exercise above.

2. Whilst inhaling and exhaling slowly, circle your fists anti-clockwise ten times and then clockwise ten times.

Neck exercises

These exercises are useful not just for people with OA or RA of the neck or shoulders, but also for anyone who carries tension in these areas. They can be performed whilst sitting or standing. Make sure your back is straight and your neck and shoulders are relaxed.

1. As you inhale, slowly tilt your head back, looking up at the ceiling. As you exhale, slowly drop your head forward, resting your chin on your chest. Repeat five times.

2. Inhaling and exhaling gently, very slowly make big circles with your head to the left five times, allowing your chin to touch your chest and the back of your head to tilt right back. Repeat, circling the head to the right.

3. As you inhale, slowly tilt your head to the left, as though you are trying to touch your shoulder with your ear. Exhale as you return your head to an upright position. Repeat on your right side.

Knee circles

This exercise loosens the knee joints, helping to prevent joint problems and improve movement in those with OA or RA of the knees.

1. Stand up straight with your neck and shoulders relaxed and legs together.

2. Bend your knees slightly, then lean forward and place your hands on your knees.

3. Move your knees in a circular motion ten times in an anticlockwise direction and then ten times in a clockwise direction, whilst inhaling and exhaling slowly.

Foot and hand circles

This exercise helps to improve flexibility in the wrists and ankles and wards off stiffness.

1. Lie flat on the floor.

2. Raise your arms so that they are at right angles to your body.

3. Raise your legs so that they are at right angles to the rest of your body.

4. Simultaneously circle both your hands and feet ten times in a clockwise direction. Then circle them in an anticlockwise direction.

The triangle

This posture helps to keep the hips and back mobile.

1. Stand up straight, with your feet together and your arms relaxed at your sides. Tuck in your bottom, lengthen your neck and tuck your chin in slightly.

2. Separate your feet so that they are about one metre apart.

3. Inhale and lift your arms to shoulder height, palms facing down and fingers outstretched.

4. Keeping your head, trunk and hips facing forward, turn your left foot outwards with the heel in line with the arch of your right foot.

5. Breathe out, then bend sideways to the left, sliding your left hand down your left leg and allowing it to rest on the shin. Stretch your right arm straight up with the palm facing forwards.

6. Make sure your legs are straight and your head and trunk are in line with your hips and legs. Breathe in and slowly turn your head to look at your right hand.

7. Come out of the posture by lifting your trunk, with your arms still outstretched. Repeat on your right side.

Take yoga classes

The best and probably most fun way to learn yoga is to attend classes run by a qualified teacher. Make sure you tell your teacher about your condition so that he or she can advise you on how to adapt the postures according to your individual needs. To find a class near you, go to the British Wheel of Yoga's website: www.bwy.org.uk. Or, if you'd prefer to teach yourself at home, visit www.abc-of-yoga.com, a site which shows you how to do the various postures using animated clips. For details of other useful websites offering further information and guidance about yoga and yoga products, see the Directory.

Safe yoga

When practising yoga at home, always proceed gently and avoid forcing an arthritic joint into a posture. Always stop if you feel any discomfort. The British Wheel of Yoga warns RA sufferers not to exercise when their joints are inflamed. Wear lightweight, loose clothing to allow you to move freely and no footwear, as yoga is best performed barefoot. Use a non-slip mat if the floor is slippery. Don't attempt inverted postures if you have a neck or back problem, or have high blood pressure, heart disease or circulatory problems. If in doubt, consult your GP first.

Chapter 7

Living with Arthritis

The pain and stiffness of arthritis can make everyday life difficult. In a recent survey of 232 people with RA by the National Rheumatoid Arthritis Society, nearly half said that being able to function physically was a top priority. This chapter looks at how to make life easier by protecting your joints, adapting your home and using helpful equipment and gadgets. There are also suggestions on how to drive, work and travel more comfortably.

38 Protect your joints

When performing everyday tasks, there are various things you can do to avoid unnecessary strain on your joints and increased pain.

- View pain as a sign that you are overdoing things – if you feel pain, take a break from whatever you are doing.

- Use labour-saving devices to reduce the amount of effort you have to use.

- Avoid gripping objects tightly – padding items like pens, toothbrushes and knives helps to relieve the strain on the thumb and finger joints and the knuckles.

- Use your bigger, stronger joints when carrying out tasks. For example, use your hip or shoulder instead of your hand to shut a door or drawer.

- Hold bigger items close to your body when you carry them.

- When lifting, use both hands to spread the load over more than one joint.

- Where possible, shift rather than lift – use a trolley to move things around in the house and a wheelbarrow in the garden.

- Avoid positions that put strain on one particular joint. For example, stand squarely to ensure your weight is supported equally by both knees.

- Instead of cleaning your whole house in one go, clean one or two rooms each day.

- You can also avoid unnecessary strain on your joints by making adaptations to your home environment and using helpful equipment.

Pace yourself

Use a weekly planner to schedule in activities using a traffic light system. Mark those activities you find easy and pleasurable with a green highlighter pen, those you find a little more taxing with a yellow pen and those you find difficult and tiring with a red pen. You can then make sure you don't have too many 'red' and 'yellow' activities on the same day.

39 Adapt your home

You may find some of the following tips helpful, depending on which of your joints are affected by arthritis and on the severity of your symptoms.

- Place the items you use the most within easy reach.
- If you have problems with balance, have handrails fitted around your home.
- Fit a handrail on both sides of your staircase for extra support when going up and down.
- If you have difficulty getting up and down stairs, consider having a stairlift fitted.
- Have lever taps fitted, instead of the type you have to turn, or fit devices called 'tap turners' to taps.
- If you find bathing difficult, consider installing a walk-in bath, or take a shower instead.

40 Use helpful equipment

Occupational therapists can advise you on changing how you do things to protect your joints and provide information about suitable equipment and adaptations to your home.

To try out a range of independent living equipment and products, visit your local Disabled Living Centre. These are run by Assist UK – see the Directory.

For information about local suppliers and service providers that loan or sell equipment, contact your local Disability Information and Advice Line (DIAL) – see the Directory.

You may also be able to borrow equipment from your local social services department or your local hospital.

Depending on your level of disability, you could also be eligible for direct payments which enable you to pay for your own care and support, including equipment. Contact your local council for more information.

Below is a list of ways you can use everyday equipment to help minimise pain and strain associated with arthritis:

- Use kitchen gadgets that make everyday tasks easier, e.g. a rubber cap gripper, kitchen knives and vegetable peelers with large or padded handles, and an electric tin opener and food processor (see Useful Products).

- If your fingers are too swollen and painful to peel vegetables, buy them ready prepared. Frozen vegetables are also a convenient alternative to fresh ones and often contain more nutrients.

- Place potatoes or other vegetables in a colander when cooking them in a pan. When they are cooked, lift them out in the colander – this saves lifting heavy pans to drain them.

- Use long-handled sponges for washing up. However, if you have stiff fingers, placing them in warm water may be therapeutic.

- Sit on a kitchen stool when preparing meals.

- Use lightweight mugs, pans and kettle.

- Buy plastic crockery if you find the normal kind too heavy.

- Fill the kettle by using a lightweight plastic jug, using just enough water for your needs.

- Buy long-handled tools with a gripping mechanism, known as reachers, to retrieve items that are further than an arm's length away.

- Use a feather duster to dust hard-to-reach areas.

- Use 'push on' clothes pegs, rather than those with a spring mechanism.

- Use a lightweight, hand-held vacuum cleaner to clean upholstery and stairs.

- Use fitted sheets that don't need to be tucked in.

- Use a trolley to move items from room to room.

- Use a long stick with a rubber end for pushing the buttons on the television and microwave.

- If you find squeezing shampoo and conditioner bottles problematic, buy empty soap dispensers, fill them with shampoo or conditioner, then label.

41 Work more comfortably

Working with arthritis can be difficult, depending on your level of disability. However, employment not only improves your financial position, but can also boost your physical and emotional well-being.

The Disability Discrimination Act (DDA) states that employers must not discriminate against a disabled person in the workplace and covers a range of issues including recruitment and the provision of appropriate facilities to enable you to do your job. Not everyone with arthritis is covered by the DDA: according to the act, a disabled person is someone with 'a physical or mental impairment which has a substantial and long-term adverse effect on their ability to carry out normal day-to-day activities'.

You would be covered if you have significant mobility problems, loss of function in one or both hands, chronic pain or difficulty lifting heavy objects because of arthritis. If the act applies to you, you have the right to 'reasonable adjustments' to help you carry out your job. Even if you are not considered disabled, it is still good practice for your employer to adapt to your needs. These adaptations could include:

- Flexible working – this might mean being able to start and finish work later, if your symptoms are worse in the mornings. You may be able to work from home and also have time off for medical treatments and physiotherapy.

- Changes to your work environment – this could include improving accessibility to your work area, providing special equipment or making adaptations to tools, adapting work furniture, or modifying your job role.

If you work at a desk, there are a number of steps you can take to reduce pain and discomfort:

- Watch your posture – sit up straight to avoid unnecessary joint strain.

- Adjust your chair so that your feet are flat on the floor.

- Your keyboard should be at the same level as your elbows and your computer screen should be positioned so that you're looking straight ahead and not having to twist your neck or shoulders.

- If arthritis affects your hands, ask for a wrist rest, ergonomic keyboard and a trackball mouse, which is easier to operate and can reduce strain.

- If finger stiffness makes typing difficult, ask for a keyboard guard – this makes it harder to hit the wrong key and also provides a platform on which you can rest your hands.

- If you use a telephone frequently, you could ask for a telephone with large push buttons and a hands-free headset.

- Get up from your desk and walk around at least once an hour.

- If you are not sure whether your workspace is suited to your needs, ask your employer to check that it complies with health and safety regulations. An occupational therapist can advise you on suitable changes and devices to help you do your job.

Sit correctly

Sir Robin McKenzie, a physiotherapist who specialises in spinal problems and is the author of *Treat Your Own Neck* and *Treat Your Own Back* (see the Helpful Reading section for details), claims that poor sitting posture is the most common cause of neck and back pain and that once spinal problems have developed, poor posture will exacerbate them.

He says that slouching in a chair makes our head and neck protrude, which overstretches the ligaments and causes distortion of the discs and leads to pain. He recommends sitting upright, with the lower back slightly hollowed – preferably using a lumbar roll for support (see Useful Products) – and keeping the upper back, neck and head straight, with the chin slightly tucked in.

If you spend long periods sitting, and especially if you have arthritis in your neck and/or spine, try the following exercises recommended by Sir Robin five or six times every hour.

Head retraction

Head retraction involves sitting and looking straight ahead, whilst slowly pulling your head backwards as far as you can, keeping your chin tucked in. Hold for a few seconds and then relax. Repeat five or six times.

Neck extension

For the neck extension, hold your head in the retracted position, then lift your chin up and tilt your head backwards as far as you can, whilst looking up at the ceiling. Remain in this position and turn your head about 2 cm to the left and then to the right. After a few seconds return to the starting position.

Simple neck stretch

This exercise was recommended to me by a qualified chiropractor. Sitting upright, slowly tilt your head towards your left shoulder, whilst dropping your right shoulder slightly. Next tilt your head to the right, dropping your left shoulder. Repeat on each side several times. To increase the stretch, place the hand from the side you are stretching towards on the other side of your head and press gently.

42 Travel without pain

With a little thought and forward planning, travel need not cause problems. The tips below will help you to travel without making any pain, stiffness or other symptoms worse.

Ten top travel tips

1. If you have mobility problems, inform your travel operator before you book, so that they can ensure your needs are met, for example by checking that your resort and hotel are easy to access.

2. If your mobility problems are severe, consider using a specialist travel company that provides holidays that are geared to your needs (see Directory).

3. Choose lightweight luggage with wheels and pack as few items as possible, to avoid having to carry a heavy load.

4. Make sure you pack essential medications in your hand luggage.

5. Be prepared for a possible flare-up whilst you're away – ensure you pack items you usually rely on to help you cope, such as a relaxation tape or your favourite massage oil.

6. To avoid overdoing things, allow yourself plenty of time to reach the station or airport at the beginning and end of your trip.

7. Midweek travel is likely to be less crowded, which means there will be less queuing.

8. Reserve an aisle seat on a bus or plane to make it easier for you to get up and stretch your legs and do simple arm stretches to reduce joint pain.

9. Take travel cushions or pillows for extra support and comfort (see Useful Products).

10. Take time differences into account when taking your medications.

Three tips to make driving more comfortable

1. Try using a wide car key holder to make it easier to turn on the ignition.

2. Wear thin driving gloves to enhance your grip on the wheel.

3. Place a silk scarf on your car seat to make it easier to twist around when getting in and out.

43 Help your child cope with arthritis

According to Arthritis Care, around 12,000 children in the UK under the age of 16 have some form of arthritis. Being diagnosed with arthritis during childhood can be particularly difficult to deal with, as arthritis tends to be viewed as something that older people have. Children and young people with the condition may feel isolated – especially if it prevents them from taking part in sport or even just playing outdoors. As well as having to deal with the pain and disability arthritis can bring, they may also have to cope with the effects it has on their appearance; in Arthritis Care's *Breakout* guide (an online resource written by young arthritis sufferers to share their experiences of the condition), 25-year-old Rionah McNichol describes how she felt self-conscious about the way she looked because her bottom jaw didn't grow normally, as a result of having arthritis.

Apart from ensuring that your child takes any prescribed medications regularly, eats a balanced diet and takes regular exercise, there are other steps you can take to help your child to cope with living with arthritis.

Promote learning about juvenile arthritis

Helping your child to learn about their arthritis will make it easier for them to understand why they feel the way they do and to be less afraid of the condition. The main arthritis organisations have produced a range of resources that both you and your child may find useful:

- Arthritis Care offers a printable online booklet aimed at children with arthritis aged seven and under, called *A Day With Sam*. Written by the parent of an eight-year-old girl called Samantha, who developed juvenile arthritis when she was just 13 months old, *A Day with Sam* is a story that aims to answer the questions a child with the condition might ask, using simple, easily understood language. Arthritis Care also publishes an informative magazine for young people with arthritis called *No Limits*.

- Arthritis Research UK has produced a booklet aimed at four- to eight-year-olds called *Tim has Arthritis* that is available as a printed copy or to download online. With the aid of colourful cartoons, the booklet explains what juvenile arthritis is and outlines the diagnostic tests and treatments a child with the condition might experience. The charity also offers a booklet called *Arthritis: a guide for teenagers* that covers a wide range of topics affecting teenagers with juvenile idiopathic arthritis. It is available in printed form, or as a PDF online.

- The Children's Chronic Arthritis Association and the National Rheumatoid Arthritis Society also offer up-to-date information about juvenile arthritis. Learning about arthritis will also make it easier to talk to others about it.

Encourage your child to talk about their arthritis

Your child may find it difficult to tell others about their illness, but you can explain that, if they do talk about it, people will find it easier to understand them and their condition and be more aware of when to offer help and support. Suggest that it may help if they have a 'rehearsed speech' that they use when someone asks them what is wrong with them, or when they feel that it is the right time to reveal that they have arthritis. It could explain a little about the illness and how it makes them feel. For example: 'I have juvenile idiopathic arthritis. It's a type of autoimmune disease that affects all of my joints and muscles and makes me feel achey and really tired.'

Children and young people with arthritis may feel depressed about having to deal with constant pain, and frustrated by the limitations that the condition imposes on them. Encouraging your child to talk openly about their feelings to you, family members, friends and teachers will help them to cope with their condition. It's also worth contacting organisations that offer workshops, group meetings and online forums where your child can share their feelings with other sufferers, such as the Children's Chronic Arthritis Association, Arthritis Care, the National Rheumatoid Arthritis Society and Youthhealthtalk (see the Directory).

Help your child to cope with arthritis at school

Coping with arthritis at school can be difficult. Children with arthritis may be absent from school a lot and may find it hard to catch up with their work. Even when they are able to attend school, they may find that symptoms such as pain and fatigue make it difficult for them to focus on their work. They may be unable to participate fully in PE lessons and even getting from one class to another may pose a problem. They may also experience bullying, which is another reason why it is important to encourage your child to communicate openly about their life and their feelings.

Preparing for university

If your child has arthritis and is interested in going on to higher education, Arthritis Care offers a useful factsheet called *Preparing for University* to help them find the university best suited to their needs.

Speak to your child's teacher

It's important that your child's teacher is kept fully informed about your child's condition, so that they can offer support and understanding. In the *Breakout* guide, Rionah McNichol says that she was lucky because her secondary school was very supportive, to the extent that they even adapted her timetable so that she could stay in the same classroom all day and be with her friends.

If you or your child's teacher/s feel that his or her progress at school is being hampered by arthritis, you or the school can request a statutory assessment of special educational needs (SEN). In this assessment, many factors, including evidence from the school regarding your child's progress and both your and your child's views, will be taken into consideration. If a statement of SEN is issued, your child will be entitled to extra help. For example, this might mean the provision of a laptop computer and printer, so that they don't have to struggle with gripping a pen, or a taxi to get to and from school if they find using public transport difficult.

> ### A guide for teachers
>
> If your child's teacher expresses an interest in learning more about juvenile arthritis, you could mention the downloadable guide for teachers called *Chat 2 Teachers*, from Arthritis Care, which aims to promote understanding of the needs of pupils with the condition.

Help for parents

Being the parent of a child or young person with arthritis can be stressful. Not only do you have to deal with the shock of the initial diagnosis, but you also have to cope with the additional demands your child's illness places on you – such as frequent trips to the GP and hospital and looking after them when they are unwell. You might benefit from talking things through with your partner or other family members. It might also help if you can speak to other parents who are in the same situation as you. The Children's Chronic Arthritis Association offers a support network to parents of children with arthritis, including telephone contact and group meetings. Arthritis Care recently launched an online parent support group called Parents Online. The UK charity Contact a Family offers a family support service and peer support from volunteer parent representatives, to help families caring for disabled children up to the age of 19.

There is also a range of literature aimed at the parents of children with arthritis; a useful book called *Kids with Arthritis – A Guide for Families* by Carrie Britton, is available free of charge from Arthritis Care. *The Chat (children have arthritis too) Guide for Parents*, which is aimed at the parents of children newly diagnosed with arthritis, is available online from Arthritis Care. *Chat 2 Parents*, aimed at the parents of teenagers with arthritis, is also available on the website. Arthritis Research UK offers a useful online guide for parents of children with arthritis, called *When Your Child Has Arthritis*.

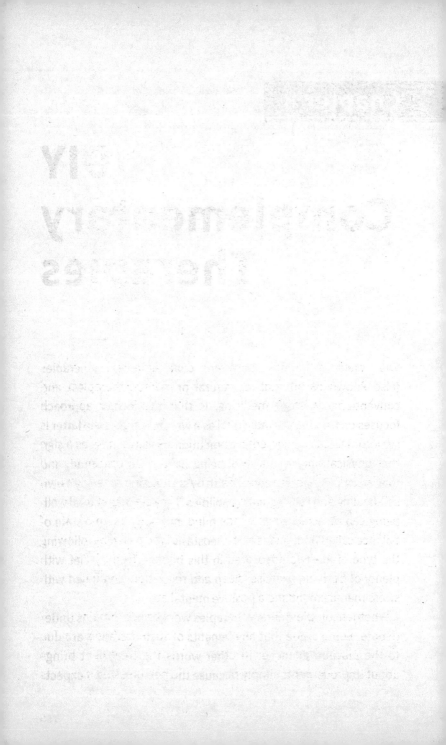

Chapter 8

DIY Complementary Therapies

The main difference between complementary therapies (also known as alternative, natural or holistic therapies) and conventional Western medicine, is that the former approach focuses on treating the individual as a whole, whereas the latter is symptom led. Complementary practitioners view illness as a sign that physical and mental well-being have been disrupted, and they attempt to restore good health by stimulating the body's own self-healing and self-regulating abilities. They claim that total well-being can be achieved when the mind and body are in a state of balance called homeostasis. Homeostasis is achieved by following the type of lifestyle advocated in this book: a healthy diet with plenty of fresh air, exercise, sleep and relaxation, combined with stress management and a positive mental attitude.

Whether complementary therapies work or not remains under debate. Some argue that any benefits of such therapies are due to the placebo effect, or in other words the treatment brings about improvements simply because the person using it expects it to, rather than because it has any real effect. However, it could be argued that, unlike drug treatments, which are comparatively recent, complementary therapies like aromatherapy, massage and reflexology have stood the test of time, having been used to treat ailments and promote well-being for thousands of years. The use of complementary therapies alongside conventional medicine received an unexpected boost recently when NICE recommended acupuncture and chiropractic treatments, along with exercise therapy, for the treatment of lower back pain. Relevant useful organisations are listed in the Directory at the end of the book.

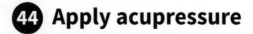 Apply acupressure

Whilst no research appears to have been done regarding the effectiveness of acupressure for the treatment of arthritis symptoms, acupuncture is widely viewed as an effective form of pain relief and there is evidence that it helps OA of the knees. Animal studies suggest it has an anti-inflammatory effect. Like acupuncture, acupressure is part of traditional Chinese medicine and is often described as 'acupuncture without needles', as it works on the same points on the body. Acupuncture also resembles acupressure in that it is based on the idea that life energy, or qi, flows through channels in the body known as meridians. An even passage of qi throughout the body is viewed as vital to good health. Disruption of the flow of qi in a meridian can lead to illness at any point within it. The flow of qi can be affected by various factors, including stress, emotional distress, diet and environment.

Qi is most concentrated at points along the meridians known as acupoints. There is some scientific evidence that stimulating particular acupoints can relieve pain. Using the fingers and thumbs to apply firm but gentle pressure to these points stimulates the body's natural self-healing abilities. Muscular tension is relieved and the circulation boosted, thereby promoting good health. The application of pressure also seems to stimulate the production of endorphins and enkephalins (pain-relieving hormones). Many Chinese people use acupressure to self-treat a range of common conditions. You can try the following simple acupressure techniques for yourself:

Beam Hill (ST 34)

To ease knee pain, use the thumbs of each hand to work on the 'beam hill' acupoints, which are situated two thumb widths above the outer edge of the kneecaps. First use gentle, circular movements and then apply firm pressure. Go to www.all-about-acupuncture.com/stomach-acupuncture-points to see a diagram showing the position of this acupoint.

Leg Three Li (ST 36)

Applying pressure to the 'three mile point' acupoints is also thought to relieve knee pain. To locate these acupoints, first find the bumps below the outer edge of each kneecap, then find the point three finger-widths down. Use each thumb to make circular motions and then apply firm pressure. These acupoints are also commonly used to treat disorders of the immune system, such as RA. Again, go to www.all-about-acupuncture.com/stomach-acupuncture-points to see a diagram showing the position of this acupoint.

Shoulder Well

To ease stiff, painful shoulders, use your middle fingers to press gently on each side of the neck on the 'shoulder well' acupoints.

These are located on the shoulder muscle halfway between the base of the neck and the end of the shoulder muscle. For an online image of this acupoint, go to www.modernreflexology.com

45 Improve your posture with the Alexander technique

The Alexander technique is a useful discipline for arthritis sufferers to learn, as it aims to improve posture and enable the body to function with the minimum amount of strain on the joints and muscles. The technique was devised by Frederick Matthias Alexander, an Australian actor, in the 1890s, when he realised that his bad posture was affecting his performances. A study published in the *British Medical Journal* in 2008 concluded that practising the Alexander technique provided significant long-term benefits for people with chronic back pain.

According to practitioners, poor posture affects bone alignment and puts unnecessary stress on the joint, ligaments and muscles. The Alexander technique focuses on restoring the correct positioning of the head, neck and back – 'the core' of the body. To ensure that you adopt the correct posture, it's important that you learn the Alexander technique from a qualified teacher. A teacher will assess your posture and movement and show you how to correct any bad habits. You will learn how to perform everyday tasks, such as turning on a tap, with the minimum of force, to help to minimise strain on the joints and muscles. Once you have become proficient, you will be able to practise yourself at home. The eventual aim is that you will naturally maintain the correct stance at all times.

46 Use aroma power

Essential oils are extracted using various methods from the petals, leaves, stalk, roots, seeds, nuts and even bark of plants. Aromatherapy is based on the belief that, when scents released from essential oils are inhaled, they affect the hypothalamus. This is the part of the brain that governs the glands and hormones, altering mood and lowering stress. When used in massage, baths and compresses, the oils are also absorbed through the bloodstream and transported to the organs and glands, which benefit from their healing effects. Since arthritis flare-ups can be linked to emotional stress, aromatherapy may be worth trying, both as a preventative measure and during a flare-up. Arthritis Research UK states on its website that 'Many people with chronic pain do report that an aromatherapy massage gives several weeks' relief'.

Patricia Davis, author of *Aromatherapy: An A–Z*, suggests that various essential oils can help to alleviate arthritis symptoms by helping the body get rid of toxins, thereby easing pain and stimulating the circulation. The oils she recommends include cypress, fennel, ginger, juniper, lavender, lemon, marjoram and rosemary.

Cypress
Cypress oil is derived from both the cones and leaves of the cypress tree and has a distinctive 'woody' smell. It both detoxifies and stimulates the circulation when added to a bath or used in massage.

Fennel
Fennel comes from the same plant family as aniseed – hence its aniseed-like aroma. The oil is extracted by crushing the seeds of the

fennel plant. It is thought to prevent the build-up of toxic waste in the body. Sprinkle in the bath, or use it in massage. Caution: fennel oil should not be used by people with epilepsy, as it may induce fits.

> ### Massage oil
>
> In massage you can generally use a two per cent dilution: this equates to two drops per teaspoon of carrier oil, although stronger oils may need more dilution. A carrier oil can be any vegetable oil, including good-quality olive or sunflower oil from your kitchen. Almond, sesame seed or grapeseed oils are equally good. Never apply aromatherapy oils to broken skin. Buy the best-quality oils you can afford; like most things, you get what you pay for – cheaper oils may not be as pure as more expensive ones.

Ginger

Ginger oil has a warming effect on the skin, which improves circulation. It can also help to ease the pain of arthritis when it is applied using a hot compress or massage. Because high concentrations can irritate the skin, it is recommended that it is used in a one to one-and-a-half per cent dilution (one to one-and-a-half drops per teaspoon of carrier oil) in massage.

Juniper

Juniper oil has a turpentine-like smell. According to Patricia Davis, it is one of the best detoxifying oils, which makes it helpful for arthritis, particularly RA and gout. Add it to the bath to help your body get rid of toxic waste.

Take an aromatic bath

Fill the bath with comfortably hot water. When you are ready to get in, add six drops of essential oil (unless otherwise stated on the label). Agitate the water with your hand to disperse the oil, which will form a thin film on the water. The warmth of the water both aids absorption through the skin and releases aromatic vapours, which are then inhaled.

Lavender

Lavender oil has many properties, which makes it one of the most useful essential oils. In arthritis it is used to relieve pain and reduce inflammation. It is effective when used in a warm bath, or as a hot compress. Japanese researchers recently reported that it has the added benefit of reducing the stress hormone cortisol. Inhaling lavender oil at bedtime has been shown to improve sleep quality by 20 per cent.

Lemon

According to Patricia Davis, lemon oil reduces acidity in the body and boosts the circulation, making it especially helpful for RA and other inflammatory forms of arthritis. Lemon oil may irritate the skin, so sprinkle just three drops in the bath and add just one drop per teaspoon of carrier oil when using it for massage.

> **Make a hot compress**
>
> Add four or five drops of essential oil to a basin of hot water and soak a facecloth or small towel. Wring out the excess moisture and place on the affected area.

Marjoram

Marjoram has a warm, spicy scent. When used in massage, marjoram oil has a warming effect that eases the pain and stiffness associated with arthritis.

Rosemary

Rosemary has pain-relieving and circulation-boosting qualities. It also eases joint stiffness when used in massage, added to the bath, or used in a hot compress. Caution: rosemary should not be used by anyone with epilepsy, as it may trigger fits.

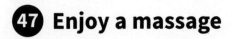 Enjoy a massage

Whenever we feel pain, we instinctively rub or massage the affected area. Massage involves touch, which can help to ease pain and stiffness and reduce stress and tension. It's thought to work by stimulating the release of endorphins (the body's own painkillers) and serotonin (a brain chemical involved in relaxation). It also decreases the level of stress hormones in the blood and improves the circulation, helping to improve the removal of toxins from the body. As the muscles relax and joint stiffness eases, mobility and flexibility improve.

Mix your own massage oil by combining eight drops of an appropriate aromatherapy oil with 20 ml (one tablespoon) of carrier oil. Ask a partner to massage the areas that are painful and stiff, or try self-massage using these basic techniques:

Stroking/effleurage – glide both hands over the skin in rhythmic fanning or circular motions.
Kneading – using alternate hands, squeeze and release flesh between the fingers and thumbs, as though you're kneading dough.
Friction – using your thumbs, apply even pressure to static points, or make small circles on either side of the spine.
Hacking – relax your hands, then using the sides, alternately deliver short, sharp taps all over.

Playing some relaxing music in the background can help to enhance the feelings of relaxation.

Safe massage

Don't massage an inflamed joint – massage around it instead to boost the circulation and relax the muscles.

48 Get help with homeopathy

Homeopathy means 'same suffering' and is based on the idea that 'like cures like' – substances that can cause symptoms in a well person can treat the same symptoms in a person who is ill. For example, bee stings can cause hot, swollen, tender swellings, so the remedy apis, which is made from bee stings, is often prescribed for arthritis sufferers with swollen, tender joints.

Symptoms like inflammation or fever are viewed as a sign that the body is trying to heal itself. The theory is that homeopathic remedies encourage this self-healing process and that they work in a similar way to vaccines. The substances used in homeopathic remedies come from plant, animal, mineral, bark and metal sources. These substances are turned into a tincture, which is then diluted many times over. Homeopaths claim that the more diluted a remedy is, the higher its potency and the lower its potential side effects. They believe in the 'memory of water', the theory that, even though the molecules from a substance are diluted, they leave behind an electromagnetic 'footprint' – like a recording on an audiotape – which has an effect on the body.

These ideas are controversial and many GPs remain sceptical. Evidence to support homeopathy exists, but critics argue that much of it is inconclusive. For example, research published in 2005 reported improvements in symptoms and well-being among 70 per cent of patients receiving individualised homeopathy. The study involved 6,500 patients over a six-year period at the Bristol Homeopathic Hospital. Critics of the studies argue that there was no comparison group and patients may have given a positive response because it was expected.

However, a systematic review of three RCTs involving 226 RA sufferers, published in the *Rheumatic Disease Clinics of North America* journal in 2000, found that those taking homeopathic remedies reported twice the benefits of those taking a placebo. Another review published in *The Clinical Journal of Pain* in 2004 concluded there was 'some evidence' that homeopathic remedies were more effective than a placebo for treating OA and RA. Other research suggests that homeopathy is better than a placebo for fibromyalgia.

There are two main types of remedies – whole person based and symptom based. It's probably best to consult a qualified homeopath who will prescribe a remedy aimed at you as a whole person, based on your personality, as well as the symptoms you experience. However, if you prefer, you can buy homeopathic remedies at many high street pharmacies and health shops.

Below is a list of homeopathic remedies, along with the arthritis-related physical symptoms and the psychological traits for which they're indicated. To self-prescribe, simply choose the remedy with indications that most closely match your symptoms. Follow the dosage instructions on the product.

Apis
Physical symptoms: Swelling and burning pain made worse by heat and improved by cold.
Psychological traits: Anxiety and restlessness.

Arnica
Physical symptoms: Acute pain, heat and inflammation associated with RA, OA and gout that are made worse by heat and continuous movement.
Psychological traits: Denial of illness.

Bryonia
Physical symptoms: Inflammation and swelling due to excess joint (synovial) fluid. The pain is worse with movement and cold weather and improves with rest.
Psychological traits: Irritability and anxiety.

Calc carb
Physical symptoms: OA with bony outgrowths on the joints. Pain that is worse first thing in the morning and after physical activity.

Psychological traits: Fear and anxiety.

Causticum

Physical symptoms: Inflammation of the joints that has led to joint deformities and joint stiffness that may be worse in cold weather.

Psychological traits: Introspection and oversensitivity.

Dulcamara

Physical symptoms: Joint pain and stiffness that is worse in damp weather and with inactivity.

Psychological traits: Impatience, irritability and restlessness.

Rhododendron

Physical symptoms: Joint pain, swelling and stiffness that are aggravated by changes in the weather and improve with warmth.

Psychological traits: Nervousness and sensitivity.

Rhus tox

Physical symptoms: Chronic arthritic pain that is worse in the morning and in cold damp conditions, but improves with heat or movement.

Psychological traits: Restlessness and agitation.

Silica

Physical symptoms: Destruction of bone and swelling near the joints. Symptoms are worse in the cold and when pressure is applied to the painful area.

Psychological traits: Lack of assertiveness, stubbornness.

Tuberculinum

Physical symptoms: Joint and limb pain, with stiffness that eases with movement and cool, dry surroundings and worsens in damp conditions.

Psychological traits: Irritability and restlessness.

Not a quick fix

Practitioners warn that homeopathy isn't a 'quick fix' – the remedies may take a while to take effect. Homeopathic remedies are generally considered safe and don't have any known side effects, though sometimes a temporary worsening of symptoms, known as 'aggravation', may take place. This is seen as a good sign, as it suggests that the remedy is encouraging the healing process. If this happens, stop taking the remedy and wait for your symptoms to improve. If there is steady improvement, don't restart the remedy. If the improvement stops, resume taking the remedy.

49 Try magnetic therapy

Practitioners of magnetic therapy claim that exposing the body to magnetic fields improves blood flow, which helps the elimination of waste products, reduces pain and speeds up healing. Some studies suggest that static magnetic fields from permanent magnets constrict and dilate the walls of capillary blood vessels, increasing blood circulation and reducing inflammation. In its information booklet *Complementary and Alternative Medicine for Arthritis*, Arthritis Research UK states that recent research has found that 'magnets can be helpful for pain, including low back and knee pain'. There are various magnetic products available, including magnetic supports for specific joints, bracelets and mattress overlays (see Useful Products).

> **Use magnets safely**
>
> Magnetic therapy is generally deemed safe, but it is not recommended if you have a pacemaker, as the magnetic field may interfere with the signal between the pacemaker and the heart. Magnets can also affect the functioning of internal defibrillators and internal insulin pumps.

50 Find relief in reflexology

Reflexology is based on the idea that points on the feet, hands and face, known as reflexes, correspond to different parts of the body (e.g. glands and organs). These are linked via vertical zones, along which energy flows. Illness occurs when these zones become blocked. Stimulating the reflexes using the fingers and thumbs is thought to bring about physiological changes that remove these blockages and encourage the mind and body to self-heal.

Practitioners believe that imbalances in the body result in granular deposits in the relevant reflex, which cause tenderness. Corns, bunions and even hard skin are all believed to indicate problems in the related parts of the body. The energy theory behind reflexology is very similar to the one underpinning acupressure, though practitioners say it is a different system. There is no reliable evidence that reflexology relieves arthritis, but there's anecdotal evidence that reflexology massage is relaxing. So at the very least, trying these techniques may relieve stress and thus lessen the frequency of your symptoms.

A reflexologist will usually work on your feet, because they believe the feet are more sensitive. However, it's usually easier to work on your hands when you are self-treating.

Neck pain relief

To relieve neck pain, use the right thumb to creep around the base of your left thumb, applying firm pressure. Repeat several times.

Shoulder pain relief

To relieve shoulder pain, use your right thumb to creep up the middle of the little finger on your left hand (with your palm facing upwards), starting from the base and finishing at the tip. Repeat several times and then perform the same movements on your right hand, using your left thumb.

Back pain relief

To relieve back pain, creep your right thumb along the whole of the spinal reflex on the left hand. This begins in the middle of the inner wrist and extends along the outside of the thumb to the tip. Repeat several times and then perform the same motions on your right hand, using your left thumb.

Recipes

This section contains recipes based on some of the dietary recommendations outlined in Chapter 3.

Roasted Vegetable Pasta (serves 4)

This recipe contains olive oil and roasted vegetables, which provide anti-inflammatory antioxidants and omega-9 (monounsaturated) fatty acids. It includes basil, which may also have anti-inflammatory properties. Note: if you like wholewheat pasta, it is preferable to the white version because it contains more fibre, so it keeps you feeling fuller for longer, which will help you to manage your weight.

Ingredients
1 red pepper
1 yellow pepper
1 green pepper
1 red onion
200 g cherry tomatoes
2 cloves garlic, crushed
4 tbsp extra-virgin olive or rapeseed oil
320 g wholewheat or white pasta
Fresh basil leaves
Sea salt
Black pepper
Grated Parmesan/Grana Padano cheese

Method

Preheat oven to 220°C/gas mark 7. Roughly chop the peppers and onions. Grease a roasting tin using a little oil. Add the chopped vegetables, whole cherry tomatoes and garlic. Drizzle with oil, lightly season and toss, to ensure all vegetables are coated. Roast in the oven for 10 to 15 minutes, until the vegetables are soft and beginning to brown. Meanwhile, add the wholewheat pasta to a pan of boiling, lightly salted water. Bring back to the boil and cook according to the instructions on the packet. Drain the cooked pasta and stir in the roasted vegetables, olive oil and torn basil leaves. Season to taste. Serve with grated Parmesan/Grana Padano cheese.

Pan-fried Spiced Mackerel with Rocket (serves 1)

This recipe contains mackerel, which supplies anti-inflammatory omega-3 fatty acids and vitamin D, as well as turmeric, which is also thought to have anti-inflammatory properties. The rocket provides antioxidant vitamins, calcium and fibre. It is also rich in folic acid (folate), which the body needs to make new cells. The action of folic acid can be affected if you are taking the DMARD methotrexate, so eating folate-rich foods may help.

Ingredients

1 mackerel fillet, cut in two
2 tsp turmeric
2 tsp smoked paprika
1 tbsp olive or rapeseed oil
50 g rocket

Method

Rub the turmeric and paprika all over the mackerel pieces. Heat the oil in a frying pan over a medium heat. Add the mackerel and fry for about two minutes on each side, until slightly golden. Serve the spiced mackerel on a bed of rocket.

Lemon and Ginger Salmon with Watercress (serves 4)

The salmon, ginger and olive oil in this dish are anti-inflammatory, while the watercress boosts iron and folic acid levels, helping to prevent anaemia, which can develop with RA and juvenile idiopathic arthritis, and low folic acid levels, which can occur in people who take the DMARD methotrexate.

Ingredients

4 skinless and boneless salmon fillets
Juice of one lemon
4 tbsp ginger, finely chopped
2 garlic cloves, finely chopped
Fresh coriander, chopped
200 g watercress
2 tbsp olive oil

Method

Preheat the oven to 200°C/gas mark 6. Place each of the salmon fillets on a piece of cooking foil. Drizzle with the lemon juice, then sprinkle evenly with the chopped ginger, garlic and coriander. Wrap the salmon fillets loosely in the foil and bake for around 15 minutes, or until the fish is cooked. Serve with the watercress, drizzled with olive oil.

Vegetable Chilli with Brown Rice (serves 4)

The vegetables in this chilli provide beneficial vitamins, minerals and fibre and, like the garlic, chilli and cumin, they have anti-inflammatory properties. Brown rice provides more fibre, vitamins and minerals than white rice and helps with weight management because it keeps you feeling fuller for longer.

Ingredients

2 tbsp olive or rapeseed oil
1 medium onion, chopped
1–2 cloves garlic, crushed
1 tsp cumin seeds
1–2 tsp chilli powder
1 butternut squash, cubed
1 celery stick, chopped
2 cans of chopped tomatoes
100 g fine green beans, cut in half
2 cans of kidney beans
320 g brown basmati rice
Fresh coriander

Method

Heat the oil in a large pan and fry the onion, garlic, cumin seeds and chilli powder together until the onions are soft and golden. Add the butternut squash, celery and chopped tomatoes, then cover and simmer for 25 minutes. Meanwhile, bring a pan of lightly salted water to boil and add the rice. Bring back to the boil and cook according to the instructions on the packet. Add the green beans to the chilli, cover and simmer for a further 5 minutes. Add the kidney beans and simmer for a further 3 minutes. Serve with the brown rice and garnish with the coriander.

Baked Bananas with Yogurt and Honey (serves 4)

In this recipe, the bananas provide anti-inflammatory vitamin C, iron and soluble fibre, whilst the natural yogurt contains bone-building calcium.

Ingredients
4 large, unpeeled bananas
4 tsp runny honey
500 g natural set yogurt

Method
Preheat the oven to 200°C/gas mark 6. Place the bananas on a baking tray and bake for 20 to 25 minutes, until the skins are blackened but not split. Put each blackened banana on a plate. Split open and top with a dollop of natural yogurt. Drizzle with a teaspoon of honey and serve.

Gingered Fresh Fruit Salad (serves 4)

The fruits in this recipe provide vitamins and minerals and are anti-inflammatory, as is the ginger. The yogurt provides calcium.

Ingredients
500 g mixed fresh fruit such as strawberries, grapes, kiwis, apple, pear (all peeled and cubed)
200 ml orange juice (freshly squeezed, or from a carton)
2 cm cube of ginger root
Natural set or Greek yogurt

Method
Place all of the fruit into a large glass bowl. Blend together the orange juice and ginger in a food processor. Pour over the fruit and gently mix together. Serve with the yogurt.

Jargon Buster

Listed below are the meanings of words and phrases that might be used when describing the diagnosis, prevention and treatment of arthritis.

Acute – something that starts suddenly and is soon over. RA is a long-term condition with acute flare-ups.

Antioxidants – substances that can neutralise free radicals. The body produces its own antioxidants but antioxidants in the diet, such as the vitamins A, C, and E, are thought to help destroy excess free radicals.

Autoimmune disease – any condition where the body produces antibodies that attack normal tissue.

Cartilage – a tough yet flexible connective tissue.

Enzyme – a protein that speeds up a chemical reaction in the body.

Free radicals – substances produced in the body following exposure to stress, sunlight and pollutants (e.g. cigarette smoke, food additives and chemicals), which are believed to cause tissue damage, or disease.

Gout – a type of arthritis affecting mainly small joints that is caused by a build-up of uric acid in the body.

Inflammation – a natural response by the immune system to irritation, infection or injury. Symptoms include redness, heat, swelling and pain.

Joint – a point where two bones meet. Some are mobile, such as the knees and elbows, whilst others are immobile, such as those between the bones in the skull.

Leukotrienes – substances produced in the body that are involved in the immune response.

Metabolism – chemical reactions in the body, such as the breaking down of food to turn it into energy.

Osteoarthritis (OA) – a condition generally caused by wear and tear of the joints that leads to pain, stiffness and inflammation.

Placebo – an inactive substance given to study participants either to compare its effects with those of a treatment or so that they can benefit from believing they have received a treatment.

Prostaglandins – chemicals produced in the body from fatty acids, some of which reduce inflammation and some of which promote it.

Randomised controlled trial (RCT) – study where participants are randomly placed in a treatment group or a control group. The treatment group receives the treatment under scrutiny, whilst the control group may receive a placebo or another treatment for comparison purposes.

Rheumatoid arthritis (RA) – an autoimmune disease, meaning it is caused by the immune system mistaking normal tissues for foreign invaders and attacking them.

Rheumatoid factor – an antibody that most people with RA have in their blood.

Selective serotonin reuptake inhibitor (SSRI) – a type of antidepressant drug that increases levels of serotonin (the 'happy hormone') in the brain.

Synovial membrane – a thin tissue around the joints that secretes a fluid that lubricates the joints and tendons to allow easy movement.

Topical – a treatment that is applied externally.

Uric acid – substance produced when proteins are metabolised in the body.

Helpful Reading

Austin, Denise, *Pilates for Every Body: Strengthen, Lengthen and Tone Your Body* (Rodale, 2002). A useful guide to Pilates with various routines lasting five or ten minutes, including one for beginners.

Black, Octavius and Bailey, Sebastian, *The Mind Gym: Give Me Time* (Time Warner Books, 2006). This book shows you how to reduce stress and use your time wisely by striking a balance between work and play and doing things that engage you and give you a sense of purpose.

Britton, Carrie, *Kids with Arthritis – A Guide for Families* (CHOICES for Families of Children with Arthritis, 2003). A comprehensive guide to juvenile arthritis that uses the experiences of children to offer insight into what it is like to live with the condition, or with someone who suffers from it. Useful reading for anyone involved in the care of a child with juvenile arthritis.

Campbell, Dr Giraud, W. *A Doctor's Home Cure for Arthritis: The Bestselling, Proven Self-treatment Plan* (Thorsons, 2002). This is an updated version of Dr Campbell's original book that was published in the early 1970s. Although some of Dr Campbell's theories are controversial, many people claim to have been helped by his eating plan, so if your symptoms are severe and are not responding to your current treatments, I believe it is worth reading this book. Overall, the diet is nutritionally sound and cutting out processed foods may well be beneficial for anyone suffering from arthritis.

Cannon, Professor Christopher and Vierck, Elizabeth, *The Complete Idiot's Guide to the Anti-Inflammation Diet* (Alpha, 2006). A useful guide to foods that contribute to inflammation and those that reduce it.

Carlson, Richard, *Don't Sweat the Small Stuff… and It's All Small Stuff: Simple Ways to Keep the Little Things from Taking Over Your Life* (Mobius, 1998). This book offers some effective strategies to help you achieve inner calm.

Davis, Patricia, *Aromatherapy: An A–Z* (Vermilion, 2005). A comprehensive guide to essential oils and how to use them to reduce stress and improve your health.

Ewin, Dr Jeannette and Patten, Marguerite, *Eat to Beat Arthritis: Over 60 recipes and a self-treatment plan to transform your life* (Thorsons, 2001). Marguerite Patten based these recipes on Dr Giraud W. Campbell's dietary programme for arthritis, after finding that it relieved her arthritis symptoms. The book includes a diet plan developed by nutritionist Dr Jeannette Ewin, which incorporates new nutritional information and builds on Dr Campbell's original guidelines.

Hills, Margaret, *Treating Arthritis Diet Book* (Sheldon Press, 2006). After suffering from arthritis as a young woman, the author developed her own 'acid-free' diet cure. This book contains recipes, including starters, main courses and desserts that she advocates for arthritis sufferers.

Hills, Margaret, *Treating Arthritis: The Drug-Free Way* (Sheldon Press, 2006). This book outlines Margaret Hill's drug-free method of treating arthritis.

Holford, Patrick, *Say No To Arthritis* (Piatkus, 1999). This book contains dietary guidelines, including advice on detecting food intolerances, as well as more general advice on arthritis. Whilst some of the author's ideas are controversial – for example, he recommends cutting out foods from the nightshade family, such as tomatoes, potatoes (except sweet potatoes and yams), aubergines and red, green and yellow peppers – the book does contain some sound advice and I believe it is worth reading.

Margo, Sammy, *The Good Sleep Guide* (Vermilion, 2008). This book is written by a physiotherapist and includes some good advice on how to select the right pillow and mattress for you, to help ensure a comfortable night's sleep.

McKenzie, Robin, *Treat Your Own Back* (Spinal Publications New Zealand Ltd, 2006). This book contains useful advice on how to manage back pain by correcting your posture and practising exercises designed to improve mobility and relieve pain.

McKenzie, Robin, *Treat Your Own Neck* (Spinal Publications New Zealand Ltd, 2006). This book is well worth reading if you suffer from neck and shoulder pain: it contains lots of helpful advice on how to avoid neck pain by improving your posture, and how to treat it through a series of exercises designed to restore mobility and relieve pain.

Useful Products

Below is a list of products and suppliers of products that may help to ease the symptoms of arthritis. The author doesn't endorse or recommend any particular product and this list is by no means exhaustive.

Atrogel Arnica Gel
Made from arnica flower tincture, which has an anti-inflammatory effect. Quickly absorbed and fast-acting.
   Website: www.avogel.co.uk

Avoca ASU Bone & Joint Health
A supplement that contains avocado/soybean unsaponifiables (ASU), non-shellfish glucosamine and methylsulfonylmethane (MSM).
   Website: www.nutramaxlabs.com

A. Vogel Stinging Nettle Urtica Drops
A tincture containing organically grown stinging nettle leaves and root. The adult dosage is 20 drops twice daily in water.
   Website: www.avogel.co.uk

Baldwins Essential Oils
A comprehensive range of good-quality essential oils.
   Website: www.baldwins.co.uk

Biofreeze Pain Relieving Gel

A range of topical pain-relieving products containing Ilex, a herbal extract from the South American holly. Available as a gel, roll-on or spray. Eases pain within minutes and the effects last up to six hours.

Website: www.biofreeze.co.uk

Cherrygood

Sugar- and additive-free cherry juice drink made from Montmorency cherries, which have been shown to help lower uric acid levels in gout sufferers.

Website: www.cherrygood.com

Clipper Organic Nettle Tea

Tea made from organically grown young nettle leaves.

Website: www.clipper-teas.com

First Choice Plus TENS Machine

Compact TENS unit with adjustable pulse.

Website: www.bodyclock.co.uk

Flexacil Ultra

Combines glucosamine and chondroitin with *Boswellia serrata* leaf, ginger root and horsetail leaf extracts.

Website: www.flexacilultra.com

Jointace Gel

A massage gel combining glucosamine, chondroitin with seven essential oils including ginger, eucalyptus, orange, clove and lavender. Can be used alongside anti-inflammatory drugs and NSAIDs.

Website: www.vitabiotics.com

Jointace Rose Hip & MSM

Tablets designed to help maintain joint mobility, containing 12 nutrients that may help boost joint health, including rose hip, glucosamine and chondroitin, along with MSM and ginger extracts.

Website: www.vitabiotics.com

Just a Little Thought

Online retailer selling a wide range of travel pillows and cushions.

Website: www.justalittlethought.co.uk

KOOLPAK reusable hot/cold pack

Hot/cold pack that can be heated in the microwave or cooled in the freezer to relieve muscular and joint pain and ease swelling.

Website: www.stjohnsupplies.co.uk

LitoZin

Contains rose hip to help maintain healthy and flexible joints and is high in GOPO. Available as capsules or powders.

Website: www.litozin.com

Magnohealth 24ct Gold Plated Magnetic Copper Bracelet

Although there is mixed scientific evidence about the use of copper bracelets, some sufferers find them helpful. This one combines pure copper with magnets, which are supposed to increase circulation and relieve pain.

Website: www.magnohealth.co.uk

McKenzie Lumbar Roll

Recommended for the prevention and treatment of back and neck pain caused by poor posture.

Website: www.mckenzieinstituteusa.org

Optiflex Glucosamine HCl 1,000 mg

Glucosamine supplement suitable for vegetarians, vegans and those with a shellfish allergy.

Website: www.healthspan.co.uk

Organic Turmeric Capsules

Ayurvedic supplement containing organic turmeric.

Website: www.pukkaherbs.com

Phynova Joint and Muscle Relief Tablets

Tablets containing extract of Sigesbeckia.

Website: www.phynovajointrelief.com

Phytodolor

Tincture containing aspen, common ash bark and goldenrod herb. Requires a prescription that is valid in the UK before it can be purchased.

Website: www.dennisthechemist.com

Pukka Active

Ayurvedic supplement containing organic turmeric, *Boswellia serrata* (Indian frankincense) and ginger.

Website: www.pukkaherbs.com

Pycnogenol

Tablets containing French maritime pine bark extract.

Website: www.healthspan.co.uk

Regenovex

Range of products for arthritis containing hyaluronic acid and green-lipped mussel extract, which are claimed to maintain the joints and aid flexibility. Includes a gel, a patch and one-a-day capsules.

Website: www.boots.com

SAMe tablets by BIOVEA

Enteric-coated (to protect from stomach acid) tablets containing 200 mg/400 mg of SAMe, vitamins B6, B12 and folic acid.

Website: www.biovea.net/uk

Seven Seas Evening Primrose Oil plus Starflower Oil

One-a-day capsules containing both evening primrose oil and starflower (borage seed) oil.

Website: www.seven-seas.com

Seven Seas Joint Care

A range of products containing omega-3 fish oil and other ingredients believed to benefit the joints, such as glucosamine and chondroitin.

Website: www.seven-seas.com

T'ai Chi for Arthritis DVD

Two-disc DVD set offering step-by-step instructions to a t'ai chi programme specifically created to help ease arthritis symptoms by Dr Paul Lam, who has himself benefited from practising the ancient art.

Website: www.taichiproductions.com

TENS Machine Direct

Online retailer specialising in TENS machines.

Website: www.tensmachines.co.uk

Tisserand Aromatherapy Pure Essential Oils

A wide range of good-quality essential oils designed to improve health and happiness.

Website: www.tisserand.com

Directory

Below is a list of contacts offering useful information and support for arthritis sufferers.

ABC of Yoga
A website offering tips, advice and poses for those who wish to practise yoga at home. Also provides meditation techniques.

Website: www.abc-of-yoga.com

Accessible Travel
A travel company that specialises in providing holidays in the UK and abroad that are specially tailored to the needs of people with disabilities.

Website: www.accessibletravel.co.uk

Arthritis Action
A UK charity founded in 1942 that aims to help people with arthritis to manage their condition, thus reducing the need for medical intervention.

Annual membership fee starts at £15. Membership benefits include access to a discussion forum, nutritional and weight management advice and subsidised therapies such as massage, physiotherapy and acupuncture, as well as a biannual magazine and self-management events.

Website: www.arthritisaction.org.uk

Arthritis Care

A UK charity that offers self-help support, a helpline service, a 'living with arthritis' forum, a bimonthly magazine called *Arthritis News* and a range of informative leaflets on arthritis. The charity also runs six-week Challenging Arthritis courses on different aspects of self-managing the condition and Local Involvement Networks, which offer sufferers the opportunity to influence local services for people with arthritis. There is also useful information to help teenagers with arthritis cope with various aspects of life, including going to school, college and university, and a free confidential helpline for children with arthritis and their parents, called The Source. Other resources include a discussion forum, online diaries written by children with arthritis and various local activities and services, such as the Young People's Project in the south of England, which offers various workshops.

Website: www.arthritiscare.org.uk

Arthritis Forum

A group and website set up by arthritis sufferers in 2005 to offer help, support and friendship to other arthritis sufferers.

Website: www.arthritisforum.org.uk

Arthritis Foundation

An American charity for arthritis sufferers that funds arthritis research and offers information and support to arthritis sufferers. The website includes the latest research into the condition, online exercise videos and an online forum where you can ask for advice from experts and learn about other sufferers' experiences. You can also sign up to a free online newsletter offering practical advice on living with arthritis.

Website: www.arthritis.org

Arthritis and Musculoskeletal Alliance

An umbrella body with 34 member organisations working in the musculoskeletal field that runs groups across the country, which aim to monitor local provision, identify and campaign on service provision issues and provide a forum for service users, planners and providers.

Website: www.arma.uk.net

Arthritis Research UK (formerly the Arthritis Research Campaign, arc)

As well as funding research, this UK charity produces a range of free information booklets and leaflets about arthritis.

Website: www.arthritisresearchuk.org

The Body Control Pilates Association

A website offering information about Pilates, a directory of qualified instructors and an online shop.

Website: www.bodycontrolpilates.com

The British Pain Society

An alliance of professionals whose aim is to advance the understanding and management of pain for patients. The website offers information on all aspects of pain.

Website: www.britishpainsociety.org

Children's Chronic Arthritis Association (CCAA)

A registered charity that offers a support network for children with arthritis and their families through 'network and area family contacts'. Also provides various educational and recreational opportunities for children with juvenile idiopathic arthritis and their families.

Website: www.ccaa.org.uk

Contact a Family

A UK charity providing advice, information and support to the parents of disabled children.

Website: www.cafamily.org.uk

Disabled Living Foundation (DLF)

A national charity that provides impartial advice, information and training on everyday living aids.

Website: www.dlf.org.uk

Handy Healthcare

A website that sells mobility aids, healthcare products and disability equipment, including a wide range of splints.

Website: www.handyhealthcare.co.uk

Health Boards

Health Boards is a US website that provides message boards where you can connect with others suffering from a range of health conditions – including arthritis.

Website: www.healthboards.com

Health Supplements Information Service

A service that aims to provide accurate and balanced information on vitamins, minerals and food supplements.

Website: www.hsis.org

Health Unlocked

An NHS site that describes itself as a 'social network for health'. You can ask questions and get answers, advice and support on a wide range of health conditions, including arthritis, from leading health organisations and online communities.

Website: www.healthunlocked.com

Helios Homeopathy

A homeopathic pharmacy with an online shop. Offers over 3,000 homeopathic remedies.

  Website: www.helios.co.uk

The Lupus Site

A website offering useful information for lupus sufferers and their families. It also hosts various forums on topics, such as living with lupus, and provides news related to the condition.

  Website: www.uklupus.co.uk

Lupus UK

A national charity offering support to people with lupus and their families. The charity has several regional groups around the UK who arrange medical talks, publish local newsletters and organise events. It also produces an informative national magazine.

  Website: www.lupusuk.org.uk

Magnetic Therapy Limited

Company specialising in magnetic products, including joint supports, jewellery, mattress overlays and pillows.

  Website: www.magnetictherapy.co.uk

The Margaret Hills Clinic

The private clinic that nurse Margaret Hills set up in 1982 in Kenilworth, Warwickshire, to help fellow arthritis sufferers recover from the disease using the holistic treatment plan she herself had developed and followed. The website includes information about the services the clinic offers, as well details of the Margaret Hills Health Food Shop, which offers a free nutritional advisory service.

  Website: www.margarethillsclinic.com

Medicines and Healthcare products Regulatory Agency (MHRA)

A government agency responsible for ensuring that medicines and medical devices work and are acceptably safe.

Website: www.mhra.gov.uk

National Ankylosing Spondylitis Society

A charity that offers information and support to AS sufferers and helps to fund research into the condition. The society has a network of over 90 centres in the UK that provide weekly exercise sessions supervised by a physiotherapist. They also sell a DVD with various exercise programmes and advice from a physiotherapist.

Website: www.nass.co.uk

National Association for Special Educational Needs (nasen)

An organisation that aims to promote the education, training, advancement and development of all those with special and additional support needs in the UK.

Website: www.nasen.org.uk

National Rheumatoid Arthritis Society (NRAS)

The National Rheumatoid Arthritis Society offers support and information for people with RA and juvenile idiopathic arthritis, their families, friends and carers, as well as health professionals with an interest in RA.

Website: www.nras.org.uk

Pain Relief Foundation

Produces information leaflets and audiotapes about pain relief. Visit the website, email or send a stamped, self-addressed envelope to their address, specifying your particular pain problem.

Website: www.painrelieffoundation.org.uk

Patient UK Experience

A forum run by Patient UK that 'lets you read about and share experiences, and post medical images', and a website that offers 'comprehensive health information as provided by GPs and nurses to patients during consultations'. The medical conditions covered include various types of arthritis and their medications, treatments and services.

Website: www.patient.info/forums

The Society of Teachers of the Alexander Technique (STAT)

Provides in-depth information about the technique and lists teachers, workshops and courses.

Website: www.alexandertechnique.co.uk

The Stress Management Society

The Stress Management Society is a non-profit-making organisation dedicated to helping people tackle stress.

Website: www.stress.org.uk

Yoga Abode

An online magazine and community for yoga fans. It offers technical advice on yoga postures and yoga products, as well as a directory of yoga classes, workshops and retreats.

Website: www.yoga-abode.com

Yoga 2 Hear

A website offering CD and MP3 hatha yoga class downloads, suitable for all levels and abilities, including a free taster session.

Website: www.yoga2hear.co.uk

Youthhealthtalk

A website where young people can watch video clips of other young people with health conditions (including arthritis) talking about their experiences. There is also a forum where young people can discuss their experiences.

Website: www.youthhealthtalk.org

IBS

A self-help guide to feeling better

Wendy Green

Foreword by Dr Nick Read,
chair of The IBS Network

IBS
A self-help guide to feeling better

Wendy Green

£8.99
Paperback
ISBN: 978-1-84953-807-7

In this easy-to-follow book, Wendy Green explains how food intolerances, gut infections and bacterial imbalance, and stress and hormones contribute to IBS and offers practical advice and a holistic approach to help you deal with the symptoms, including simple dietary and lifestyle changes, and DIY complementary therapies. Find out 50 things you can do today to help you cope with IBS, including:

- ▶ Identify your IBS triggers and learn how to manage them
- ▶ Choose beneficial foods and supplements
- ▶ Manage stress and relax to reduce flare-ups
- ▶ Discover practical tips for living with IBS
- ▶ Adopt preventative strategies
- ▶ Find helpful organisations and products

Menopause

A self-help guide to feeling better

Wendy Green

Foreword by Janet Brockie, menopause nurse specialist,
John Radcliffe Hospital, Oxford

Menopause
A self-help guide to feeling better

Wendy Green

£8.99
Paperback
ISBN: 978-1-84953-823-7

Do you think you might be going through the menopause? Are you confused by conflicting advice about HRT? Or are you unsure which natural alternatives are effective? In this easy-to-follow book, Wendy Green explains common physical and psychological symptoms and offers a holistic approach to help you deal with them, including simple dietary and lifestyle changes and DIY complementary therapies. Find out 50 things you can do today to help you cope with the menopause, including:

- ▶ **Ease hot flushes and reduce the risks associated with menopause**
- ▶ **Learn the truth about HRT and make informed choices**
- ▶ **Discover how to beat middle-aged spread and look younger**
- ▶ **Find helpful organisations and products**

Have you enjoyed this book?
If so, why not write a review on your favourite website?

If you're interested in finding out more about our books, find
us on Facebook at **Summersdale Publishers** and follow us on
Twitter at **@Summersdale**.

Thanks very much for buying this Summersdale book.

www.summersdale.com